Using YOGA TH
to Promote
MENTAL HEALTH in
CHILDREN and ADOLESCENTS

HANDSPRING
PUBLISHING

EDINBURGH

Using YOGA THERAPY to Promote MENTAL HEALTH in CHILDREN and ADOLESCENTS

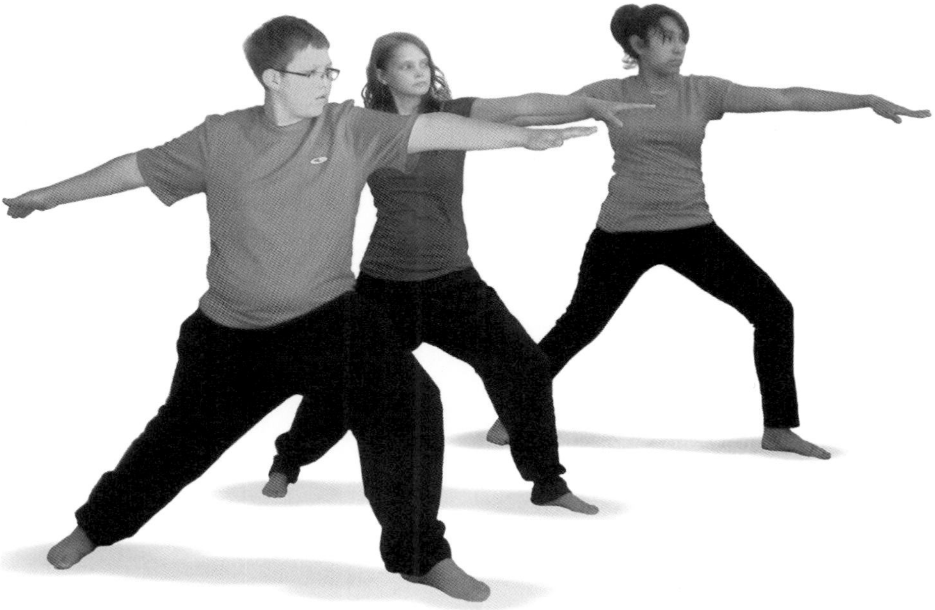

Michelle J FURY
MA, LPC, RCYT
Yoga Therapist, Ponzio Creative Arts Therapy Program,
Children's Hospital Colorado

HANDSPRING PUBLISHING LIMITED
The Old Manse, Fountainhall,
Pencaitland, East Lothian
EH34 5EY, United Kingdom
Tel: +44 1875 341 859
Website: www.handspringpublishing.com

First published 2015 in the United Kingdom by Handspring Publishing Limited

ISBN 978-1-909141-19-3

British Library Cataloguing in Publication Data
A catalogue record for this book is available from the British Library

Library of Congress Cataloguing in Publication Data
A catalog record for this book is available from the Library of Congress

Commissioning Editor Sarena Wolfaard
Copy editing by Katja Abbott
Design direction and cover design by Bruce Hogarth, kinesis-creative.com
Front cover photo: Randall Streiffert, Children's Hospital, Colorado
Author photo: Laurie Callahan, Rendition Studios, www.renditionstudios.com
Project Management by Nora Naughton, NPM Ltd.
Index by Laurence Errington
Typeset by DiTech Process Solutions, India
Printed by Bell and Bain Ltd. Glasgow.

The
Publisher's
policy is to use
paper manufactured
from sustainable forests

TABLE OF CONTENTS

Foreword		*vii*
Preface		*ix*
Introduction		*xiii*
Chapter 1	Adaptations for Developmental Stages	1
Chapter 2	Chronic Pain	11
Chapter 3	Emotion and Behavioral Regulation	21
Chapter 4	Yoga Therapy for Symptoms of Trauma	37
Chapter 5	Eating Disorders and Body Image Issues	51
Chapter 6	Suicidal Ideation and Non-Suicidal Self-Injurious Behaviors	63
Chapter 7	Psychosis	75
Chapter 8	Yoga Therapy for Sensory Integration Issues	81
Chapter 9	Practice Library	87
References		113
Appendix		121
Index		125

FOREWORD

Using Yoga Therapy to Promote Mental Health in Children and Adolescents is not only a guide to strategies that have been created and tested through trial and error, but a harbinger of changes to come in public health. This is a groundbreaking summary of work that will only continue to grow.

The rise of mental and behavioral health problems in children in the United States, and in much of the western world, is unprecedented. In the United States today, over one in every three youths will have a significant mental health problem before they turn 18 years of age (Costello et. al., 2003). Visits to both pediatric primary care settings and pediatric emergency departments for mental health problems have increased markedly in recent decades, and now account for up to 25% to 50% of primary care and 5% of pediatric emergency department visits (Chun et. al, 2013). Clearly, there are more children in the United States with mental health problems than can be treated with traditional medical services.

While the pathogenesis of mental health problems is still poorly understood, we do have some evidence for risk factors. Genes that are associated with higher risk are slowly being identified, but each of these at best explains a small percentage of the variance. Genes and environment interactions may be one key to understanding the causes of mental health problems, but genes do not mutate or change so quickly as to explain the large increase in prevalence of mental health problems. Rather, it is likely that changes in the environment are the salient risk factors for increased prevalence of these disorders. Environmental influences include *in utero* toxic exposures and stressors, early life traumas and losses, socio-economic disadvantage, and family dysfunctions (Copeland, 2009). The numbers of these risk factors present in childhood are reliably associated with increased rates of mental health problems across the lifetime (Dube et al., 2001.).

Where, then, does yoga therapy for youth fit in? The types of environmental precipitants of poor mental health are ubiquitous, most children and youth are exposed to them in some form, and they are difficult to undo. The hope for yoga therapy is that it may provide children with a strategy to help them cope better with the stressors in their current environment, as well as potentially reverse some of the maladaptive stress responses of their physiological system. Yoga, practiced regularly, improves the hypothalamic-pituitary-adrenal (HPA) response to stressors, which is tied to a variety of chronic mental and physical disorders such as depression, diabetes and heart disease (Sharma, 2014). Yoga therapy promotes a state of mindfulness, which has been scientifically shown to improve adult mental health (Hoge et. al., 2013). While there are a number of interventions to teach and promote mindfulness, the age-old mind and body awareness teachings of yoga have much to offer in enticing youth into a more mindful state.

As Michelle Fury so aptly describes in this book, traditional yoga starts with the teaching of codes for living – correct behavior and attitudes, which is helpful for youth who have not been otherwise given this structure in their life. The yoga path then continues with the learning of physical postures, practices that are often fun and engaging for children, but also strengthen the body, teach discipline, and develop endurance. Many children progress to learn how to control the breath, and with this practice lessen their physiologic arousal, fear states, and bouts of depression. Children become more mindful with each of these steps, and as they advance they become more and more comfortable with deep relaxation as well as meditation.

It is no wonder then, that, as prior Chair of the Department of Psychiatry and Behavioral Sciences at a large academic children's hospital, I was delighted to welcome yoga therapy into the "toolbox" of strategies we use to help children struggling with mental health problems. We are fortunate to have two yoga therapists, and have incorporated yoga therapy into all of our clinical programs, from acute inpatient care through routine outpatient care.

Michelle Fury has had the longest and most varied clinical yoga experience with children and teens in our psychiatry programs. She has developed her own wisdom from years of engaging with youth who bring a variety of challenges to yoga. Michelle has exercised creative persistence coaxing these youth into trying yoga and helping them progress in the practices. I have been amazed to see how she has led many of them to successes through yoga.

It is truly my joy and pleasure to introduce this book, full of wise strategies gleaned by Michelle during her many years of working with our patients. I hope that from it, yoga therapists and yoga teachers will learn ways in which to engage psychologically challenged youth in this healing path, and help them to mitigate the multitude of stressors that contribute to their problems. The need is high, the chance of success is great, and the time has come for integration of yoga into child mental health treatment.

References

Chun, T. H., Katz, E. R., & Duffy, S. J. (2013) Pediatric mental health emergencies and special health care needs. *Pediatric Clinics of North America*. 60(5). p. 1185–1201.

Copeland, W., et al. (2009) Configurations of common childhood psychosocial risk factors. *Journal of Child Psychology and Psychiatry*. 50(4). p. 451–459.

Costello, E. J., et al. (2003) Prevalence and development of psychiatric disorders in childhood and adolescence. *Archives of General Psychiatry*. 60(8).
p. 837–844.

Dube, S. R., et al. (2001) Childhood abuse, household dysfunction, and the risk of attempted suicide throughout the life span: findings from the Adverse Childhood Experiences Study. *Journal of the American Medical Association*. 286(24).
p. 3089–3096.

Hoge, E. A., et al. (2013) Randomized controlled trial of mindfulness meditation for generalized anxiety disorder: effects on anxiety and stress reactivity. *Journal of Clinical Psychiatry*, 74(8)
p. 786–792.

Sharma, M. (2014) Yoga as an alternative and complementary approach for stress management: a systematic review. *Journal of Evidence-Based Complementary & Alternative Medicine*. 19(1). p. 59–67.

Marianne Z. Wamboldt, MD, RYT
Professor of Psychiatry and Pediatrics
University of Colorado, School of Medicine

PREFACE

At the time of writing this book, plenty of interest exists in pediatric yoga's therapeutic benefits for children and adolescents (Galantino et al., 2008; Birdee et al., 2009; Kaley-Isley et al., 2010), yet there is no higher education degree in yoga therapy for children and adolescents (at least not in the United States). Research suggests that yoga may be beneficial for a number of pediatric issues, including behavioral symptoms (Galantino et al., 2008; Birdee et al., 2009; Kaley-Isley et al., 2010), but there are currently no publically available, evidence-based approaches. The relatively new field of yoga therapy is only starting to recognize that its therapeutic use for mental health is a different branch to its therapeutic use for more physically rehabilitative needs. As a result, one of the goals of this book is to articulate and systemize an approach to pediatric yoga therapy for mental health that both clinicians and researchers can use and build upon.

To illustrate the benefit of yoga therapy for mental health, meet a former patient I'll call "Jarod." Jarod wrote me a card when he discharged from treatment to share what yoga therapy meant to him, "(Yoga) has shown me that I can have a powerful effect on others. But most importantly it showed me how to find some happiness within myself" (personal communication, 2012). I'd seen Jarod for individual yoga therapy while he was in treatment for an eating disorder the summer after he'd graduated from high school. Jarod said he'd been teased as a kid for being overweight, until he started playing baseball and working out regularly. His love of the game, combined with the praise he received for losing weight, fueled him to lose more and more weight. What had started as a healthy impulse turned into an eating disorder when his need for others' approval outweighed his body's needs. The words from his letter echo a 2009 *Time* magazine article that said yoga can "empower people while priming them to access their deepest emotions" (Kornfeld, 2009).

Like Jarod, other young people can benefit from yoga therapy as a tool to achieve optimal mental well-being. Currently, there is a global concern regarding the mental health of children as well as adults. The World Health Organization has delivered a standardized survey (called the World Mental Health Survey, or WMH) in 28 countries to determine the prevalence of mental health issues. In a 2009 report on the WMH survey, Ronald Kessler and associations found that the "WMH analyses show that early-onset mental disorders are significant predictors ... of a larger pattern of associations between early-onset mental disorders and a wider array of diverse life course outcomes that might be conceptualized as societal costs" (p.30).

People today want options in their approach to physical and mental wellness. Treating mental health issues exclusive of physical ailments, or vice versa, has lost traction in the public eye. In 2009, the Centers for Disease Control in the United States found that a large portion of people sought complementary and alternative (CAM) methods of medical treatment either instead of or in addition to allopathic medical care. A recent Google search for "mind body practices" yielded approximately 23 million results. Given this number, it is not surprising that Western medicine has begun to embrace the public's demand for CAM care. The fact that my job, and the team I work with, exists is a testament to this demand.

Since 2006 I have provided yoga therapy services at Children's Hospital Colorado in the Pediatric Mental Health Institute. My position is part of the Ponzio Creative Arts Therapy Program, which includes yoga, dance/movement, music and art therapies. Like my colleagues, I am a licensed psychotherapist who works in collaboration with the other mental health staff (such as psychologists, psychiatrists and social workers) to provide integrative care for the children and adolescents we serve.

This combination of allopathic and complementary medicine is called Integrative Medicine (IM). In the IM approach, a team of clinicians work together to provide care for individual patients. For instance, part of my job entails working on the Integrative Headache Clinic in the Outpatient Neurology Clinic for adolescents with chronic headache. Along with traditional allopathic interventions like medication and nursing, we provide yoga, nutrition and psychological services to our patients.

My own interest in yoga as therapy for the pediatric population extends beyond my professional role. I started practicing yoga as a young adult in college. I'd just changed my major to psychology because others told me I was a good listener. But while I excelled at listening to others, much like Jarod I didn't know how to listen to my own needs. I grew up looking after my older brother, who was diagnosed with Tourette's Syndrome, learning disabilities and hyperactivity in the late 70's before educators knew much about any of these complex neurological and behavioral problems. He also suffered from migraines. The lack of understanding about my brother's condition meant he spent a lot of time in the principal's office, and not much time getting the treatment and care he actually needed. Because I observed my brother receiving a lot of negative attention, I focused on getting good grades and staying out of the way. When someone recommended I try yoga, I acquiesced but didn't expect much. Yet the moment I learned to practice *ujjayi* breath while holding yoga poses, I was hooked. I could concentrate in three-hour college classes with a sustained attention previously foreign to me, and I developed a new self-confidence. I learned how to listen to myself. Yoga taught me how to be aware of the present moment in a way that felt incredibly healing to me.

Starting yoga in my early adulthood while also studying psychology made it clear to me that yoga and mental health go hand in hand. Perhaps it is because I was introduced to yoga when I was just becoming an adult myself that I saw a natural connection between the two. But I am not alone. Parents and health providers alike are looking for non-pharmaceutical ways to help their children and adolescents cope with our stressful, fast-paced world. Given that today's children are tomorrow's adults, and given the current mental health crisis we seem to be in presently, it makes sense to empower our young people with a tool like yoga that costs nothing, but increases in value as children practice and enter adulthood themselves.

References

Anon., 2012. Thank You. [letter] (Personal communication, 2 Aug. 2012).

Birdee, G.S. Yeh, G.Y., Wayne, PM., Phillips, R.S., Davis, R.B. & Gardiner, P. (2009) Clinical applications of yoga for the pediatric population: a systematic review. *Academic Pediatrics*. 9 (4). p. 212–220.

Galantino, M.L., Galbavy, R. & Quinn, L. (2008) Therapeutic effects of yoga for children: a systematic review of the literature. *Pediatric Physical Therapy*. 20. p. 66–80.

Kaley-Isley, L.C., Peterson, J., Fischer, C. & Peterson, E. (2010) Yoga as a complementary therapy for children and adolescents: a guide for clinicians. *psychiatry*. 7 (8). p. 20–32.

Kessler, R.C., Aguilar-Gaxiola, S., Alonso, J., Chatterji, S., Lee, S., Ormel, J., Usten, T.B., & Wang, P.S. (2009) The global burden of mental disorders: an update from the WHO World Mental Health (WMH) surveys. *Epidemiologia e Psichiatria Sociale*. 18 (1). p. 23-33.

Kornfield, A.B.E. (2009) *Psychotherapy Goes from Couch to Yoga*. [online] Available from: http://content.time.com./time/health/article/0,8599,1891271,00.html [Accessed 2 December 2013]

Michelle Jeanne Fury
Denver, Colorado, USA

April, 2015

DEDICATION AND ACKNOWLEDGMENTS

Dedication

This book is dedicated to my big brother, Tony. It is also dedicated to three of my greatest teachers—Shannon, Abbii and Bren. I am still learning from you and our time together.

Acknowledgments

The word *sangha* in Sankrit means community. I have been held in the support of a sangha *par excellence* while writing this past year. As you read it, I hope you feel the care and humor that they each brought to this endeavor.

Thank you to my readers, who painstakingly helped me keep each chapter on course: Sarena Wolfaard, Barb Gueldner, Kristen Ramsey, Marianne Wamboldt, Sita Kedia, Erica Viggiano, Robin Gabriels, Louise Goldberg, Mindy Solomon, Elizabeth Easton and Kelly Birch. Thank you to Tia Brayman, for your hard work and expertise in all things jpeg and graphic design.

Thank you to my teachers, who infused in me the joy of learning and the confidence to share what I know with others: Richard Freeman, Sheri Vanino, Cindy Lusk, Jeanie Manchester, Jamie Turner Allison, MacAndrew Jack, Jeffrey Price, Abby Wills, Hansa Knox, Mahajyoti Berman and Bethann Bierer.

Thank you to my publisher Handspring Publishing, especially my commissioning editor Sarena Wolfaard and my copy-editor Katja Abbott.

Most especially thank you to my favorite English teacher Miss Anne Gibb, who gave me a motto that I share with my patients regularly, "We may not always like the things you do, but we always like you!"

INTRODUCTION

This book outlines a framework of clinical yoga therapy that addresses the whole child. I will address collections of behaviors and clinical symptoms that tend to co-occur in the children I see in my practice. This includes but is not limited to DSM-5 diagnoses, since this is the *lingua franca* of our field. Some of the categories include eating disorders, Autism Spectrum Disorder (ASD), mood disorders and trauma. In some cases the DSM-5 category is a chapter in and of itself, as is the case with eating disorders. In other cases the category is woven into a chapter. For instance, ASD is included within the chapter on sensory integration. Literature reviews are included in each chapter to orient the reader to the theoretical basis for this work. Case studies illustrate the unique and common presentations we find in day-to-day care.

As a teacher and therapist myself, I understand how important it is to have an easy reference guide when building a yoga session of any kind. As a result, each chapter ends with at least one sample practice, including simple illustrations of the poses. Sample practices are offered for age groups I see most often for a particular set of symptoms. For instance, sample practices for psychosis are offered only for the adolescent age group, since this is primarily the age group where we see symptoms of psychosis. Chapter 9 gives detailed instructions for poses illustrated and other techniques mentioned in chapter practices.

My goal in writing this book is twofold. Firstly, I will articulate the methods I use with a variety of mental health symptoms and stages of growth in children and adolescents. There is a general need in the field of CAM and IM for instructive texts like this that will help trained practitioners in medical and mental health settings to integrate yoga into their current practice. Secondly, I want to help create a methodology that can be replicated and used in research to build the evidence base for pediatric yoga therapy. I am reminded of an excerpt from Dr. Timothy McCall's groundbreaking book *Yoga As Medicine*, in which he quotes Swami Sivananda: "Yoga does not quarrel with science. It supplements science" (2007, p. 47). My greatest hope is that in these pages you will find the inspiration and resources you need to fuel your own journey of yoga therapy for pediatric mental health.

Reference

McCall, T. (2007) *Yoga as Medicine: The Yogic Prescription for Health and Healing.* New York: Bantam Dell.

Adaptations for Developmental Stages

1

"I think yoga can be so beneficial for kids!" said the yoga teacher I was touring at Children's Hospital Colorado where I work. I regularly speak with other yoga teachers like this young woman, as well as therapists or mental health clinicians who want to combine yoga and pediatric mental health. "But teaching yoga to kids is harder than it looks," she added.

"Yes, kids need different things than adults do," I agreed. Not only do children require simplified instructions for yoga poses, they need a practice that is fun and engaging to their developmental level. This means that children and adolescents at various developmental stages need different teaching styles. For instance, when I teach Bhujangasana, Cobra Pose, *to a 6-year-old I add hissing sounds. When I teach it to a 16-year-old I offer more detailed instructions (but not as many as I would to an adult) and I relate it to his athletic interests.*

As I continued talking with my young guest, we discussed what it means to add "therapy" to this equation. Though yoga itself has an innately therapeutic element to it, there is a difference between yoga and yoga therapy. Adding the pediatric component complicates the picture even further. But as this fellow yoga teacher said, there seems to be great benefit to learning yogic techniques during the child and adolescent years.

Because I receive so many requests from fellow teachers like the one mentioned above, this book is written primarily for yoga therapists and/or teachers seeking to offer therapeutic yoga services. Thus, a basic knowledge of both yoga practice and yoga philosophy is assumed. In addition, I will most often refer to the reader as *yoga therapist*, since many people reading this book will be aspiring to become yoga therapists, or offer yoga therapeutically in a clinical setting. However, this book is also written for mental health clinicians and researchers who practice yoga and want to integrate it into their clinical practice or research studies. As such, the extant (or existing) research literature is reviewed, and current psychological terms are defined and used.

What is pediatric yoga therapy?

Yoga

To fully understand the context in which pediatric yoga therapy has arisen, and how we can best use it, let's first define the terms *yoga* and *yoga therapy*. Yoga means "to yoke" in Sanskrit and is thought to be about 4 000 years old (Feuerstein, 1989). Yoga is both a set of practices and a philosophy.

One of the most important branches of yoga philosophy that informs contemporary yoga is the philosophical school of Patanjali, called *raja-yoga* (royal yoga) or *yoga-darsana* (yoga system) (Feuerstein, 1989). Around 200 BC, Patanjali wrote the first book to systemize yoga called the *Yoga Sutras* (Iyengar, 1979). Georg Feuerstein (1989) said that Patanjali's philosophy is ontological (i.e., a study of existence). Iyengar called yoga in general a "pragmatic science" (1979, p.xx). In other words, the practices of yoga can help us with the issues of our human condition, including our mental well-being.

Patanjali's philosophy bears a striking resemblance to some of the founders of Western psychology like Freud and Winnicott. One of Patanjali's main tenets is that humans' highest goal is striving to know and inhabit an experience of *purusa*, translated by Feuerstein (1989) as "root consciousness" (p. 6). Root consciousness, as described by Patanjali and expanded upon by Feuerstein, greatly resembles what Freud called "die Seele" (Bettelheim, 1982) and Winnicott referred to as the "true self" (Winnicott, 1965, p. 147). In Winnicott's view, the true self is our very "experience of aliveness" (p. 147). It is the experience of being "real" that comes from body sensations like our heartbeat and breath. Winnicott, like other object relations psychologists, said the true self is cultivated during childhood when the sense of self is developing (p. 144).

We will explore this concept of a developing sense of self, its role in mood regulation and mental health, and how pediatric yoga therapy can assist with it in Chapter 3.

Yoga therapy

According to the International Association of Yoga Therapy (IAYT), "yoga therapy is the process of empowering individuals to progress toward improved health and well-being through the application of the philosophy and practice of Yoga" (IAYT website, 2014). Georg Feuerstein further refined the definition to include the integration of "traditional yogic concepts and techniques with Western medical and psychological knowledge" (IAYT website, 2014). In his book *Yoga for Wellness* (1999) Gary Kraftsow, creator of American Viniyoga Institute and Viniyoga Therapy, refers to yoga's ability to support "optimal health." When it comes to mental health, this philosophy of optimizing health, rather than "curing" illness, is essential. Thus, central to this book's definition of pediatric yoga therapy for mental health are these three points:

- that it is individualized
- that it is an integration of traditional yogic concepts with medical and psychological knowledge
- that its purpose is to optimize health.

Pediatric yoga therapy

Niyamas: Rules of conduct for developing bodies and minds

The specialized needs of children and adolescents with regards to yoga could be considered the "rules of conduct" when teaching children as opposed to adults. In a sense, they are the *niyamas* of pediatric yoga practice. The *niyamas* are one of the eight limbs of yoga, consisting of five principles of personal conduct (Iyengar, 1979). Of the five principles, three apply most to children and yoga practice: *santosa* (contentment), *tapas* (discipline) and *svadhayaya* (study of the self). Children and adolescents are not motivated by fear or "shoulds" nearly as much as adults are. They are motivated by activities that they find fun and engaging, for example, activities in which they find contentment. Thus, a yoga therapist (or teacher) must first find those yogic practices and techniques that interest a child. Once a child or adolescent finds some contentment in yoga practice, the yoga practice itself empowers him to learn more about his body and mind. In other words, he is learning more about himself *(svadhayaya)*. Contentment and learning about himself then fuel his discipline.

The need for research

For those of us who practice and teach yoga, the benefits are self-evident. But as mentioned above, offering yoga as a therapy for children and adolescents requires understanding how to individualize and customize practice to optimize health and well-being. To that end, research provides a much-needed mechanism for determining what poses and practices are beneficial for which students.

The gold standard in the world of research is a double-blinded, *randomized controlled trial* (RCT) with large numbers of subjects. This ensures a degree of objectivity, which is made possible by a highly controlled environment. However, it is challenging to conduct RCTs on the benefit of yoga in "real life" situations like a hospital, clinical or even school setting, because so many variables are out of the researchers' control.

Some of the complaints about yoga research thus far include: 1) the trials aren't very well controlled, 2) often if there is blinding it is one-sided or not at all, and 3) recruitment issues (Evans et al., 2012; Hainsworth et al., 2013). This is not simply a function of yoga being a new topic of research. It is also a function of yoga's subjective nature. While I believe yoga will continue to present these challenges for researchers, research that provides evidence of benefits is important for creating standardized, meaningful approaches to care.

Research on the therapeutic use of yoga with children and adolescents is growing (Galantino et al., 2008; Birdee et al., 2009; Greenberg & Harris, 2011). Greenberg and Harris (2011) outlined several needs to create a viable body of research, including the quality and rigor of studies designed. This book directly addresses two other needs outlined by Greenberg and Harris (2011): 1) it uses a developmental approach to provide age-appropriate interventions, and 2) it offers clear descriptions of interventions that can be systemized and reproduced for the purpose of consistency and research.

Early intervention

One potentially promising application of yoga therapy in pediatric mental health is as an early intervention strategy. *Early intervention* is a term that describes behavioral strategies used to ameliorate signs and symptoms of a disorder (or disease) early in a child's life (*The American Heritage Medical Dictionary*, 2007). Early intervention strategies may lessen many behavioral symptoms that could later result in diagnoses like ADHD or Autistic Spectrum Disorder (ADD Treatment Centers, 2005; Rogers & Vismara, 2008). In Australia and New Zealand, Birchwood and MacMillan (1993) advocated using early intervention strategies with regards to schizophrenia. Throughout this book, we will explore how the use of yoga therapy, as part of an early intervention strategy, may help ameliorate symptoms and maximize potential for young people.

In this chapter, we will explore three developmental stages in the growth of children and adolescents. Adapting yoga therapeutically to meet the needs of children's various developmental stages requires careful consideration of five key areas: brain development and neuroplasticity, adaptations through ages and stages, the bell curve versus the individual, scope of practice of the yoga therapist, and the family system.

Childhood development and pediatric yoga therapy

A. Brain development and neuroplasticity

Brain development and neuroplasticity have enduring impacts on childhood development. Having a basic understanding of brain development and neuroplasticity allows a yoga therapist to mirror and support this development and neuroplasticity in young people. In particular, this knowledge helps one develop yoga sequences and a teaching style that match the child at his level.

Neuroplasticity refers to the fact that our brains are malleable (or *plastic*) over the course of our lifetime, especially during childhood development. As we can see in Figure 1.1, the brain literally plays an outsized role early on in our development. Perry (2009) says, "Because the

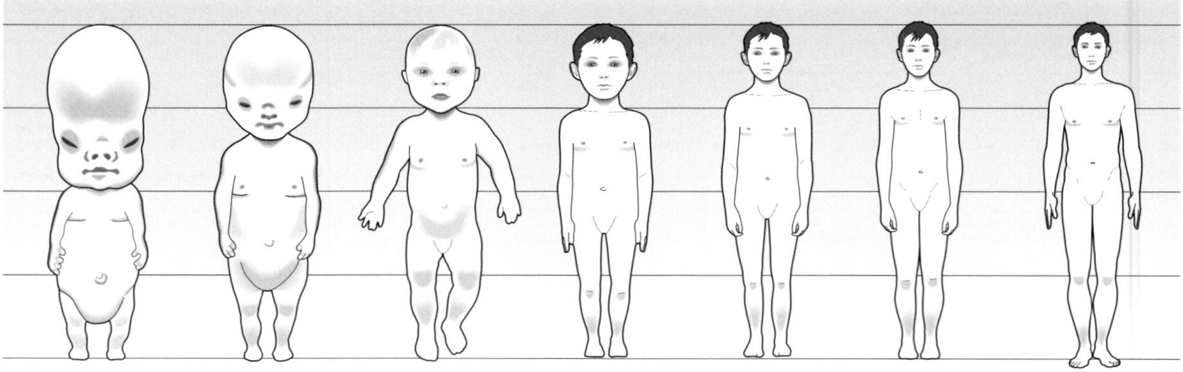

Figure 1.1
The proportions of the head and body change over the course of a child's development (Santrock, 1996).

brain is most plastic (receptive to environmental input) in early childhood, the child is most vulnerable to variance of experience during this time" (p. 245).

Yoga therapy shows a lot of promise with regards to optimizing neuroplasticity throughout life. Yoga therapist and physical therapist Neil Pearson says, ". . . one goal of Yoga therapy is to take advantage of the natural capacity for neuroplasticity" (2008, p. 79). Perry (2009) says that "somatosensory interventions that provide patterned, repetitive neural input to" children's young brains have the potential to "diminish anxiety, impulsivity, and other trauma-related symptoms that have their origins in dysregulation of these systems" (p. 243).

In normal brain development different parts of the brain develop at different times. This means that at different times in childhood, some areas of the brain may be well developed while others are not. In addition, "the developmental stage of a child has a profound impact on how an educational, caregiving, or therapeutic experience will influence the brain" (Perry, 2009). Thus, our therapeutic approach needs to match a child's current developmental needs.

The beauty of yoga is that it allows the child to become more aware of his internal experience through yogic techniques like asana, breathing and mindfulness games. The more we, as yoga therapists, understand how the brain develops throughout childhood, the more we are able to empower the child to explore in developmentally appropriate ways. For instance, if a child exhibits behavior like fast speech and hyper body movements, a yoga therapist might ask the child to imitate a snake (otherwise known as *Snake Breath*) to help the child calm himself down. Once the child's attention has been engaged and his energy has been calmed through the technique, the yoga therapist can offer other focusing or calming practices like *Balasana* (Child's Pose).

Engaging in yoga practice in this way allows the child to explore yoga techniques in ways natural to him, and then report back to us what he finds. Listening to a child's reports about his experience of doing yoga gives the yoga therapist information about

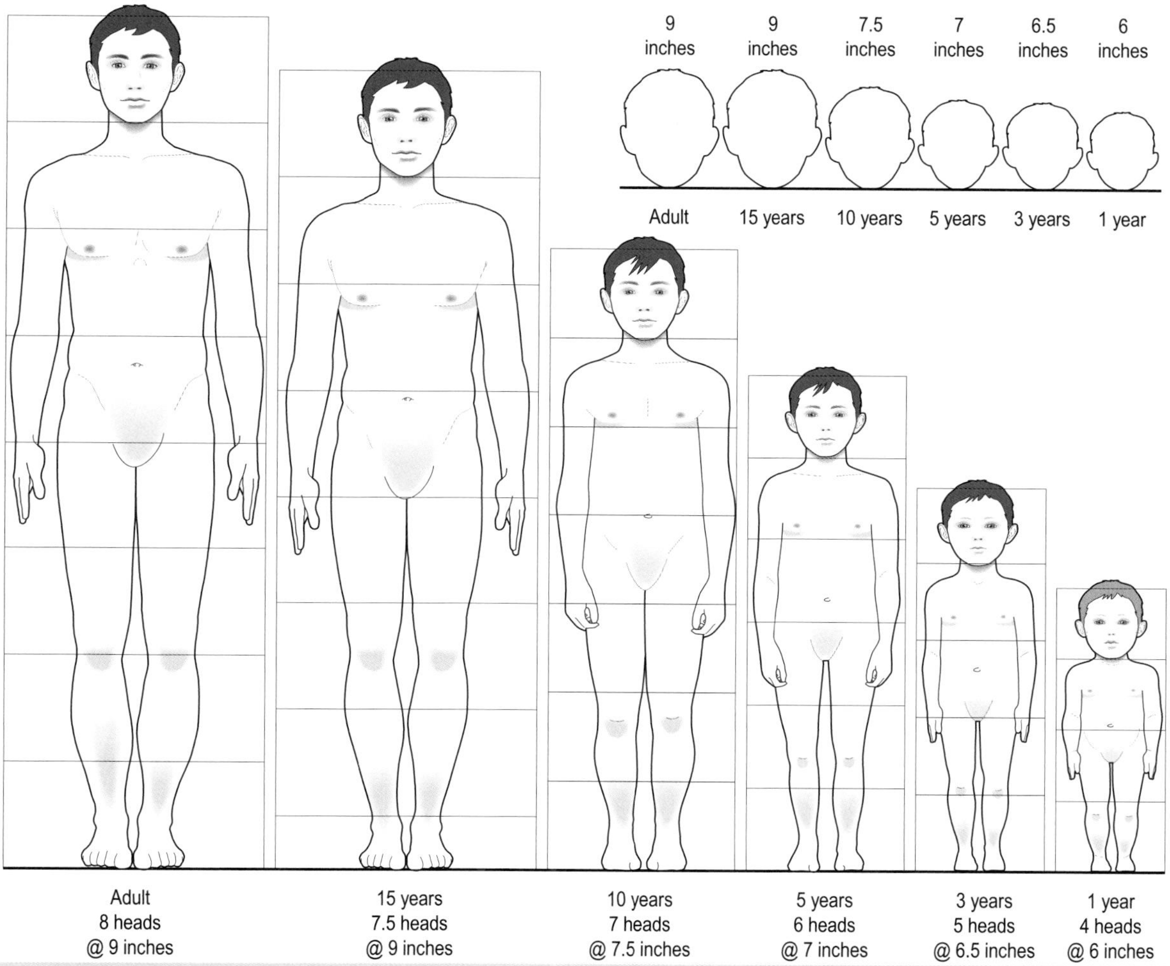

Figure 1.2
The sheer physical changes that occur over the course of childhood illustrate the need for adapting yoga poses to meet those changes and needs.

the way he thinks and experiences his world. As a result, the therapist can respond with yoga interventions appropriate to the child's stage of development in a collaborative fashion.

B. Adaptations through ages and stages

"Infants and children are not miniature adults. Body size, proportions, muscle, bone and (ligamentous) strengths are different..." (Huelke, 1998, p. 93). Figure 1.2 illustrates how different children's bodies look in relation to adults' bodies as well as to one another.

With so many internal and external changes occurring on an ongoing basis in children, it is helpful for treatment providers to have a reference guide that summarizes all of these changes. This book features three broad stages of development adapted from the *Growth and Development Summary* (1990) chart used at Children's Hospital Colorado, and are as follows: Pre-schooler (3 to 5 years), School-ager (5 to 13 years), and Adolescent (13 to 18 years). These are commonly used developmental stages in the fields of medical and mental health. By using these stages, a yoga therapist is not only able to conceptualize new cases and develop treatment plans, but can speak conversantly with other medical and mental health professionals about them.

Pre-schooler: 3 to 5 years

In the United States 3 to 5-year-olds begin schooling known as pre-school, so they are often referred to as "pre-schoolers." At this age, children lose their round babyish appearance as their arms and legs lengthen and they take on more mature proportions. They tend to have boundless physical energy for new gross motor skills, and are beginning to acquire some fine motor skills. Cognitively, their thought process is *pre-operational* (Piaget, 1973), meaning that they do not understand concrete logic yet and so their understanding is limited to the information provided in the present moment. On the other hand, they have vivid imaginations. This is how *magical thinking* comes about—i.e., believing that an occurrence in consensus reality has come about because of a fantasy in this child's mind. For instance, a child may be angry with his mother in the morning and think that the intensity of his anger has caused her to get hurt later in the day. This is also an example of *egotism*, meaning that the child believes that things happen in the world based on his thoughts and feelings.

Despite their natural egotism, children at this stage are also sensitive to others' feelings, and begin to develop a conscience. As a result, attending school helps them foster social skills and satisfy their curiosity about their ever-expanding world. This is also the perfect age to introduce children to yoga. At this age, the physical outlet of yoga helps children to harness their energy. A yoga group structured around themes like animals, elements in nature, or friendship can help them channel their energy and cultivate social skills. However, it needs to be a very loosely structured group. If the yoga group consists of mostly 3 and 4-year-olds, the group should be more like structured play. A yoga therapist working with either an individual or a group needs to be flexible and responsive to the spontaneity of this age group. For older age groups, sticking to structure is important. But for this age group, go with the flow. If your goal as a yoga therapist is to cultivate self-regulation through Balloon Breathing, and the child refuses to do it but instead stays in Tree Pose for several seconds, it's best to enthusiastically encourage the child to do Tree Pose with the other foot for a little longer. Yoga sessions for this age group should be no longer than 30 minutes, so that the children leave with a sense of mastery and accomplishment.

The purpose of yoga for this age group is not to teach specific poses but instead to cultivate a sense of playfulness and fun while also learning self-regulation. It's best to give 1 or 2-step instructions, using four to six-word sentences. Alignment instructions are moot with this, since they shouldn't be staying in poses for very long. The poses indicated for this age include poses centered on the themes noted above—animals, elements in nature, and ones that teach friendship and teamwork. Kids at this age love sound effects, so try leading a few poses that incorporate these. Sound effects are a great way to introduce breathing techniques, such as Snake Breath. Relaxation for this age group should be very short and consist of simple imagery or visualizations that encourage the use of the child's imagination. It's very important to allow time at the end of the session for children to share what they experienced or imagined to foster their social skills and budding sense of self in community.

School-ager: 5 to 13 years

Children older than 5 and below 13 years of age are sometimes referred to as "school-agers" in the US because they are in primary school. Physically, their senses are as developed as adults', but they tend to prefer the familiar over the new. For example, children at this age may become fixated on a limited diet of food they know, and refuse to try new things. This group sees steady gains in weight and height. As a result, they may experience growing pains with the stretching of muscles and the growth of long bones. This group also may experience fatigue—this is especially important for yoga therapists to be sensitive to. (A child who protests she is too tired to do yoga may simply be tired because her body is in the process of growing.) This is the age when many of us participate in organized sports for the first time, and become interested in fine motor skills like art or playing a musical instrument. Girls in the upper part of this age group may be at the beginning of puberty.

Whereas the younger age group needed license to be spontaneous, this age group thrives on structure, even when they argue to the contrary. Cognitively, they are concrete thinkers so once they know the rules they want everyone to follow the rules. They are also active, eager learners and the structured learning environment helps them focus their attention best. While children at this age now understand past, present and future they are still magical thinkers. The combination of concrete and magical thinking of this age group means they learn well through allegory and storytelling. Behaviorally speaking, school-agers are motivated by their anticipation of praise and blame.

Yoga for school-aged children can increase awareness of the internal body sensations and emotional states. Group yoga can help school-agers continue to foster crucial social skills. Limit instructions for a yoga pose to four steps. Do give alignment cues for safety, as needed. When setting limits with this age group and the previous one, use a positive spin: "If you keep your mats flat, we'll play a fun game at the end!" (Instead of saying, "Don't curl the ends of your mat up.") One of the most effective tools for creating social skills, as well as classroom management, is to invite participants to "lead" yoga poses from a set of yoga flash cards. Like their younger peers, these children also relax well with visualizations that encourage them to use their imagination, which they can now hold for up to 5–7 minutes.

Adolescence: 13 to 18 years

Adolescence is the age range in which puberty occurs, triggering established, and when a wide variety of physical development in both sexes. As a result of sizeable hormone increases, adolescents' behavior can be quite labile. The adolescent years are a time of great inner and outer turmoil. The irony is that cognitively adolescents' brains are as developed as adults', save the myelination of the cerebral cortex. *Myelination* is the process by which *neurons*, or nerve cells, are coated with a fatty substance that helps synaptic connections happen faster and allows for more complex brain processes (Frasier-Thill, 2010). As a result, adolescents tend to be very idealistic while not understanding subtleties or long-term consequences. An adolescent may look to her peer group for approval before her parents or other adults. But whether she shows it or not, she does value adults' opinions and role modeling, so it is important to give good guidance even if it seems like she's not listening.

Though adolescents are capable of doing almost all poses that adults can do, there are a number of caveats:

- Adolescents should hold poses for a shorter period of time
- they will only benefit from one or two adjustments once in a pose (their attention span is not the same as adults')
- due to individual growth patterns, yoga poses and techniques need to be individualized more for adolescents.

This is also an age when many get injured in sports, so it is important to ask about injuries before starting yoga practice. Adolescents especially love balancing poses. Unlike their younger peers, this group does not like to "lead" poses off yoga flash cards. To this group, such a suggestion will seem childish. When it comes to relaxation, this group sometimes does well with much longer relaxation practices like *Yoga Nidra*, or more intensive focusing techniques like the *Sa Ta Na Ma mantra.*

C. Bell curve versus individual

As mentioned earlier, RCTs are the gold standard of research studies. The results of such studies often give us averages or norms of all the individuals who participate. When plotted on a graph, these results look like a bell in a normal distribution—thus the term "bell curve."It is helpful to understand bell curve trends for different age groups and various diagnoses. But it is also important not to overgeneralize. Due to individual patterns of growth and development in children and adolescents, their individual needs matter a great deal.

As a yoga therapist in a pediatric hospital, I see individual children and adolescents, I facilitate groups of children of similar ages or diagnoses, and I lead multifamily groups. Whether I see a child individually or in a group, I strive to see each child for who s/he is. In the initial meeting with a child, I consider two things: the child's individual strengths and challenges, as well as the common behaviors, skills and development of a child her age.

D. Scope of practice

Understanding the limits of one's knowledge in a field is called *scope of practice*. Wikipedia defines scope of practice as a term "used by national and state/provincial licensing boards for various professions that defines the procedures, actions, and processes that are permitted for the licensed individual" (Wikipedia, 2014). While yoga therapy is not yet a licensed profession, the International Association of Yoga Therapy (IAYT) sent a memo to its members in September 2014 announcing that it is embarking on a multi-year project of creating certification guidelines for individual yoga therapists. The advantage to setting standards and creating clear guidelines of practice is that it clarifies the profession. For those who want to pursue a career in yoga therapy, standards and rules create a clear path to obtaining the necessary education, training and licensing. Even more importantly, standards and guidelines protect the consumer. In the case of pediatric yoga therapy this is especially important since the consumers are children.

While standards and scope of practice are important in any profession, they are especially important in pediatric and adolescent mental health, where creating a therapeutic rapport is critical to the success of therapy (Oetzel & Scherer, 2003). When it comes to treating mental health symptoms in children and adolescents these issues are even more central to good care. But this is also a conundrum, because getting appropriate training in a timely, affordable manner is challenging—especially when there is no clear yoga therapy track for specialty fields like pediatric mental health.

Yoga therapist Amy Weintraub (2013) offers a helpful view on how to approach this conundrum. She suggests that specialty training for either yoga therapists or mental health clinicians is preferable to more extensive requirements. In other words, it is possible for mental health professionals to offer yogic techniques without obtaining certification as a yoga teacher or therapist. It is equally possible for yoga therapists to work with individuals struggling with mental health issues. Weintraub (2013) says, "Specialty training in the aspects of yoga that are appropriate for a clinical setting is vital for the therapist's knowledge of how to apply and lead these practices safely, but training as a yoga teacher or yoga therapist is not necessary" (p. 16).

In the context of pediatric yoga therapy, scope of practice seems to boil down to three factors: the patient's acuity, the practitioner's qualifications (whether that practitioner is a yoga therapist or a mental health clinician) and institutional regulations where the practitioner offers or wants to offer services.

For those interested in pursuing a career in a clinical setting like a hospital, it is helpful to look at the kinds of jobs offered in that setting, and then get the required training for one of those jobs. Many jobs offered in a hospital setting require certification or licensing. Once an individual has obtained the training, supervision and certification or licensing required, she could then propose integrating yoga into her job. Certification and licensing in these fields provides reassurance to medical and mental health institutions that a yoga therapist has the required training and experience to work within the established medical and/or mental health system.

E. The family system

Working with children means working with their families. *Family systems theory* (The Bowen Center website, 2014) states, "Family members so profoundly affect each other's thoughts, feelings, and actions that it often seems as if people are living under the same 'emotional skin.'" The family unit is a child's first experience of *sangha*, or community, and a template for how she will interact with others in her world. In order to truly understand the "emotional skin" of a child's experience, a yoga therapist needs to work with the child's family, regardless of what form it takes. On a practical level, working with the family is essential since children are minors and therefore their parents are their legal guardians. When I see children for individual yoga therapy I invite the parent to attend either the first full session, or a portion of it. Like every child, every family is unique. I have regular check-ins with all families, but the frequency of this depends on the family. Obviously the younger the child, the more the parent is involved.

Establishing a good rapport with a child as well as his family or other support system creates a sense of trust and security among all members. If difficult family dynamics do arise, a strong relationship with the child as well as his caregivers can create an open, supportive environment for challenging family dynamics to be discussed and worked through openly.

Case study

Aidan was 8 years old when I first started working with him in a pediatric inpatient unit. Aidan is now 14, and exhibits behavior consistent with Bipolar II Disorder. (Because he is younger than 15 years of age, he is not formally diagnosed.) His mood regularly swings from depressed and irritable to manic and violent. The first time he attended my yoga group at age 8, Aidan loved the colorful yoga cards used in group, and expressed surprise at how Snake Breath and Tree Pose helped him regulate his mood. Yet he struggled to stay focused on the task at hand, and was easily distracted by peers or by his own boundless energy. With each passing week in yoga group, I noticed an improvement in Aiden's attention to task and ability to regulate his own mood. When he was discharged, Aidan told his mother he wanted to continue practicing yoga as part of his coping skills. His mother talked to his treatment team to ensure that he would continue to receive yoga when he was discharged. As a result, I saw Aidan for individual yoga therapy on a weekly basis in our outpatient clinic for about a year. Now he has a treatment plan that includes self-regulating yoga poses, a regular sleep schedule, and an effective medication regimen that help control his symptoms.

The length and nature of Aidan's yoga sessions has changed dramatically over the years. Aidan was first introduced to group yoga during his inpatient stay, where I limit sessions to 30–45 minutes consisting of 6–10 yoga asana and breathing techniques. Because the ages of children on this unit range from 4 to 12 years of age, I keep the groups short so that as much of the group as possible feels a sense of mastery and success in what is often their first experience of yoga therapy. So when I began seeing Aidan individually, we increased the time to 50 minutes, and I was able to show him poses specifically suited to his needs. During our session we would do about 30 minutes of yoga poses, sandwiched between a check-in of his progress in the beginning, and rewarding games and check-out at the end of the session. Now that he is 14 years old, he can do hour-long yoga sessions, consisting of 5–minutes of breathing techniques, 10–12 poses, and up to 10 minutes in deep relaxation.

In summary

As outlined in this chapter, children are moving targets when it comes to the way we develop treatment plans of yoga therapy for them. What works at one age (colorful yoga flash cards) can be ineffective at another age. Creating a systemized approach informed by childhood development models is essential for adapting our yoga interventions to children's changing needs. In addition, considering five key areas help the yoga therapist integrate the child's needs with developmentally appropriate practices. These areas are:

1 brain development and neuroplasticity
2 adaptations through ages and stages
3 the bell curve versus the individual
4 scope of practice and
5 the family system.

Chronic Pain

2

> *An eight-year-old who attended one of my outpatient yoga groups for headache pain said he couldn't believe how good he felt after his first yoga class. He said he hadn't felt this little pain in a long time. I later learned from other providers in the headache clinic that this boy and his family were very encouraged by his experience of yoga and the entire clinic.*

The physicality of yoga practice may have helped this little boy feel empowered, because he was doing something about his pain. Regardless of the reason, it is true that the physical movements of yoga practice may have relieved muscle tension that was contributing to his headache (McCall, 2007). The physical movements of yoga are called *asana* (poses or postures). *Asana* is one of the eight limbs of yoga practice, and are said to bring steadiness, health and mental equilibrium to the practitioner (Iyengar, 1979).

Yoga is a mind-body practice and as such it is a promising treatment strategy for chronic pain, because physical pain and mood go hand in hand. Mood is affected by chronic pain, and one's experience of pain is affected by mood. For instance, if we feel a lack of control we tend to experience more pain than if we feel like we're in control (Pearson, 2008). In addition, pain and psychological factors are often comorbid (Baliki et al., 2008; Pearson, 2008; Tracey, 2010; Fitzgerald, 2011; Zernikow, et al., 2012).

But there is a special twist for children and adolescents who experience chronic pain. UCLA's Pediatric Pain Program (Evans et al., 2012) concluded that the impact of pain on children and adolescents may have serious consequences: "The expectation of youth is to enjoy a full social, academic, and work life, and chronic pain and its associated disability often present barriers to such normative developmental processes. The assumption is that if left untreated, difficulties associated with chronic pain may persist or even compound across adulthood. Management of chronic pain in youth is best approached from a holistic, biopsychosocial model" (p. 269).

This statement handily summarizes a growing understanding of chronic pain in youth, and the ways in which yoga therapy may offer relief Evans and colleagues (2012) identify a trio of factors (biological, psychological and social) that contribute to the pediatric experience of chronic pain : biological, psychological and social. Pain early in life is experienced differently than in adulthood (Fitzgerald, 2011; Evans et al., 2012; Hainsworth et al., 2013), and childhood pain can have long-term effects (Fitzgerald, 2011; Evans et al., 2012; Zernikow, et al., 2012). From the biopsychosocial perspective, yoga may offer a powerful tool in combating chronic pain in youth (Evans, et al., 2012; Hainsworth et al., 2013). As a result, this chapter will explore how chronic pain impacts young people's biology, psychology and social life, and how yoga may help.

Addressing the biopsychosocial nature of chronic pain with yoga therapy

The biology of pain

Pain hurts physically. It has its origins in biology. Thus, any approach to reduce it must first address its physical origins. Yoga targets the physical sensation of pain by teaching the body to relax. Yoga helps relieve muscle tension that may contribute to the experience of pain (McCall, 2007). In the Integrative Headache Clinic (IHC) at Children's Hospital Colorado, we often see adolescents who suffer from chronic headaches due to postural issues or past injuries that have led to misalignment. McCall (2007) says yoga "can help strengthen muscles, educate the body in how to use them, and improve postural habits like holding the head forward of the spine" (p.321).

Yet the way perception of pain (also called *nociception*) arises goes beyond physical sensations, and involves our emotional, cognitive and sensory experience (Tracey, 2010). Neuroscience calls this complex neurobiological pathway the *pain matrix* (Tracey, 2010; Fitzgerald, 2011). Fitzgerald (2011) defines the pain matrix as "a complex network of cortical and subcortical brain structures involved in the transmission and integration of pain" (p. 18). Unfortunately, recent research shows that brain structures can be altered when the pain matrix is triggered, leading to the experience of chronic pain even after the initial physical injury is resolved (Baliki et al., 2008; Pearson, 2008; Tracey, 2010; Fitzgerald, 2011; Evans et al., 2012).

The psychology of chronic pain in youth

When it comes to young people and chronic pain, the neurobiological and psychological intersect in ways that can have a deleterious and enduring impact on their lives. Fitzgerald (2011) says that the assumption may be that children and adolescents are "catastrophizing" their pain when in actuality their brains have been altered through the pain matrix to experience pain more readily than before the injury. Thus, children and adolescents who experience pain often and early in life may be primed neurologically to continue experiencing pain throughout their lives (Fitzgerald, 2011; Evans et al., 2012; Zernikow, et al., 2012).

Changes that occur in a child's brain due to chronic pain can lead to psychological sequelae, such as depression and anxiety. One of the ways that chronic pain seems to most negatively affect a child's mental health is through lack of control. Chronic pain takes away a child's ability to do normal activities like play outside with friends. In addition, the child is usually also subjected to medical tests, treatments and directives over which she has no say. Whereas an adult usually has some say in personal medical decisions, a child or adolescent (under the age of 15 years) may not. Yet t perception of control is key to pain management. Neil Pearson, a physical therapist and yoga teacher reviewed a study that explored subjects' perception of control over their pain. "The results showed that when subjects believed they had no control, they experienced increased pain..." (2008, p.79).

Yoga therapy empowers children and adolescents experiencing chronic pain by giving them an active way to cope with their symptoms. For this reason, I tell the adolescents attending IHC that we offer yoga therapy as a coping skill as much as for pain relief. The yoga session is 50 minutes and consists of 10 *asana* that promote relaxation and pain relief. Before and after yoga group, participants rate their level of pain and relaxation on a scale from to (with 0 being no pain or relaxation and 10 being maximum pain or relaxation).

Over the course of 18 months a retrospective chart review was conducted of 40 children and adolescents who attended IHC. While the pain scores decreased slightly, the change was not clinically significant. However the relaxation scores did increase at a clinically significant level. This small trial demonstrates that yoga may be an effective coping skill in conjunction with other allopathic interventions (like pharmacology, nursing and nutrition) for reducing chronic headache in adolescents.

Helping adolescents increase their awareness of positive states like relaxation is an important life skill, and there is growing consensus that yoga does just this (McCall, 2007; Pearson, 2008; Evans et al., 2012). Yoga's ability to increase positive emotions can reverse the physiological effects of negative emotions (Wren et al., 2010).

The impact of chronic pain on youth's social life

Chronic pain takes children and adolescents away from their peers and family at a crucial time in their social development. A frequent complaint I hear about from adolescents attending IHC is a sense of isolation. While isolation is a common feeling for anyone with chronic pain, the problem is compounded for children and adolescents who developmentally should be increasing their relations with their peers. Thus group yoga therapy offers a support system to this isolated demographic (Evans et al., 2012; Hainsworth et al., 2013). In the adolescent groups, I emphasize the peer relationships in the room. Adolescence is a time in life when we naturally gravitate to and listen to our peer group more than we do anyone else (including parents and family). Adolescent peers can be an incredible support system for one another, especially when they role model positive coping skills. I have witnessed many adolescent boys change their minds about yoga's benefits on seeing their peers' positive response to yoga poses.

Case study

"Rebecca" is a feisty, quick-witted 21-year-old who has spent most of her life dealing with the pain and sequelae of cystic fibrosis (CF). CF is a genetic hereditary, chronic disease that affects the lungs and digestive system. The body produces a thick, sticky mucus, which clogs the lungs and leads to life-threatening lung infections. It also stops the body from breaking down and absorbing food. "I've always known my life was different but I didn't think it would take this road." Rebecca was referring to the severity of her symptoms and how her innumerable hospitalizations and treatments have affected her life. Like many who suffer from chronic illness, Rebecca finds it difficult to differentiate between pain and other symptoms like breathlessness, pressure or coughing intensity. However, her pain is so severe and chronic that one of the regular members of her treatment team is a pain psychologist. Along with a host of other physical diagnoses, Rebecca is also diagnosed with depression and anxiety secondary to CF.

I first met Rebecca when she was 14 years old and had joined a study on yoga for physical and mental health issues. Being part of a yoga class with peers who also suffered from physical illnesses was a rare occurrence for Rebecca. Those with CF are both susceptible to infection, and can transmit it easily. But her doctors had determined her immune system was strong enough, and that as long as she wore a mask throughout class, she would not infect or be infected by others. The yoga study afforded Rebecca the rare opportunity to socialize with peers who also dealt with chronic pain and illness. She regularly reported

Case study *(Continued)*)

feeling more relaxed after these yoga sessions, and was one of our most enthusiastic participants.

A year after she participated in the study, she obtained a grant to pay for six yoga sessions with me. In these one-on-one sessions, Rebecca learned breathing and relaxation techniques to add to her pain management skills. I also taught her several standing balance poses that she subsequently requested regularly. Rebecca identifies as being a tomboy, and her diagnosis of CF had gotten in the way of this self-concept. When she was 10 years old she received her first metaport, a device implanted surgically that delivers food and medicine. The metaport forced Rebecca to give up sports: "It was hard because I love to run around and beat up boys...I had to sit on the side lines and watch (others), and then still be careful." Rebecca said that the standing balance poses we did in her individual yoga sessions made her feel strong, and may have reminded her of her inner tomboy.

In summary

Chronic pain affects all aspects of a person's life. But it is especially detrimental to youth who are forming their world-view based on these formative years. Evans et al. (2012) and Hainsworth et al. (2013) identified a biopsychosocial model to treat pain, using yoga therapy as a complementary practice with traditional forms of treatment for pediatric pain. Using this model, yoga therapy targets the biological aspect of pain by relaxing tense muscles, teaching proper muscle engagement and cultivating good posture. It targets the psychological aspect of children and adolescents' pain by giving them an active coping skill that empowers them to live their lives as fully as possible. It also targets the impact living with chronic pain has on young people's social lives by providing a support group of peers experiencing similar issues.

Practices for pain

General guidelines for yoga therapy for each of the three age groups listed in Chapter 1 are provided below. A sample practice is included at the end of each section. For the sake of ease, the yoga therapy suggestions assume an individual session, versus a group session. However, the techniques offered could just as easily be used during group yoga therapy sessions.

A. Pre-schoolers

(Maximum time: 20 minutes)

Children of this age haven't yet learned the difference between "good" and "bad" hurt, so anything perceived as painful can be scary and stressful for them. Thus with this age group it is best to explain things in very concrete, simple terms. Visual aids that reinforce verbal explanations are invaluable.

Pre-schoolers have vivid imaginations, so making yoga interventions playful is a must. This can include breathing practices with sound effects like Snake Breath (see Chapter 9 for full instructions). However, if breathing practices bring up more anxiety it's best to switch to a distracting practice like shaking the limbs or engaging another sense perception like smell (peppermint or lavender oil) or touch (holding a piece of ice or something soft and reassuring, like a stuffed animal).

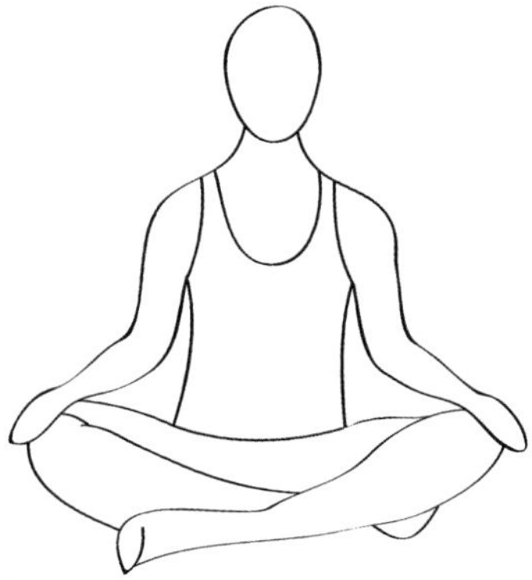

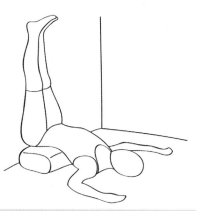

Figure 2.1
Sukhasana (Simple Sitting Pose) with Snake Breath

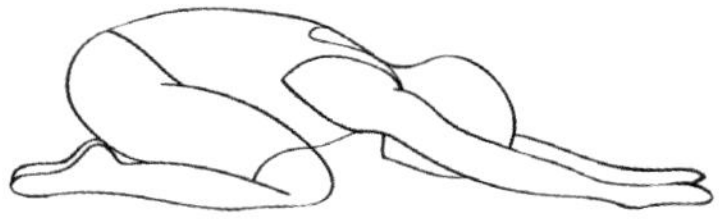

Figure 2.2
Balasana (Child's Pose)

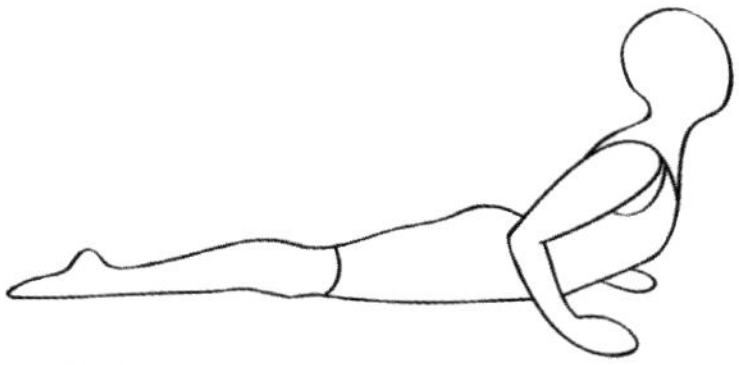

Figure 2.3
Bhujangasana (Child's Pose)

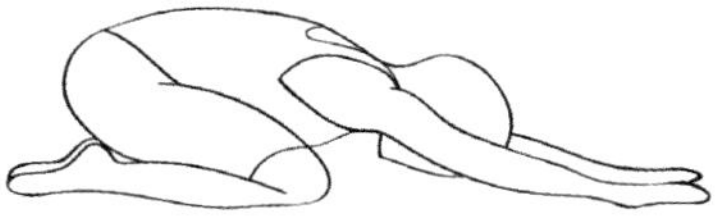

Figure 2.4
Balasana (Child's Pose)

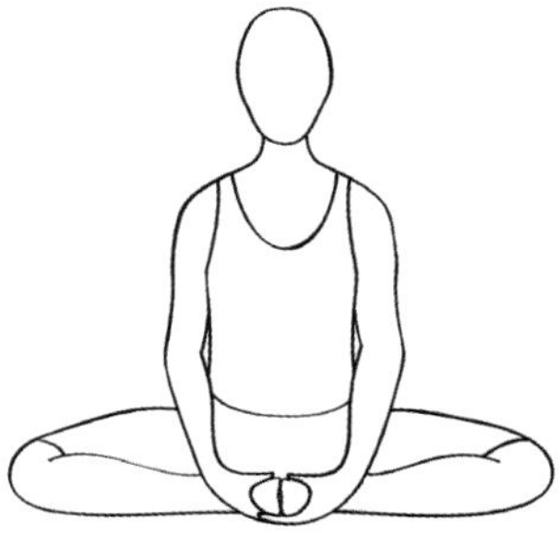

Figure 2.5
Baddha Konasana (Cobbler's Pose)

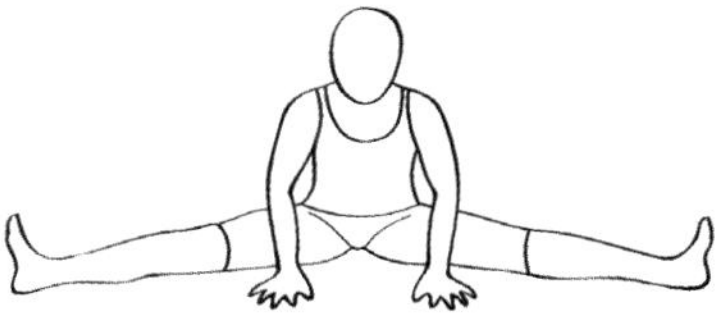

Figure 2.6
Upavistha Konasana (Seated Wide-Angle Pose)

Figure 2.7
Viparita Karani (Legs-up-the-Wall Pose)

B. School-aged children

(Time: 30–45 minutes)

Because chronic pain can take a child of this age away from his social life, inviting peers and siblings to join the yoga therapy sessions can help normalize his experience. As with the other age groups, the school-aged child may suffer from a feeling of powerlessness over the pain and the medical procedures he has to endure. After our first or second sessions I invite the child to lead some or all the poses and I encourage him to show his family and siblings, which can give him a further sense of mastery and empowerment.

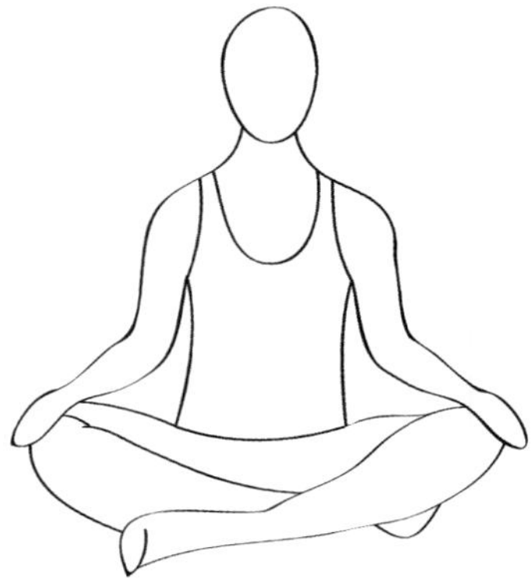

Figure 2.8
Sukhasana (Simple Sitting Pose) with Snake Breath

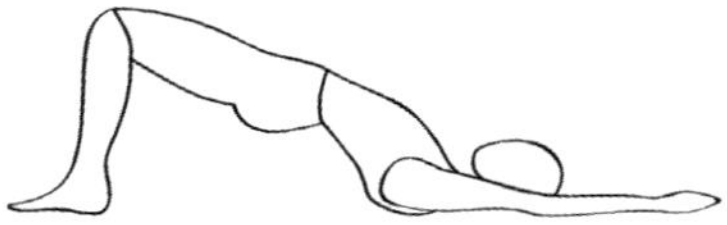

Figure 2.9
Setu Bandha Sarvangasana (Bridge Pose) Vinyasa—repeat five times

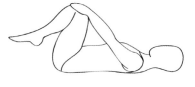

Figure 2.10
Apanasana Vinyasa—repeat 5–10 times

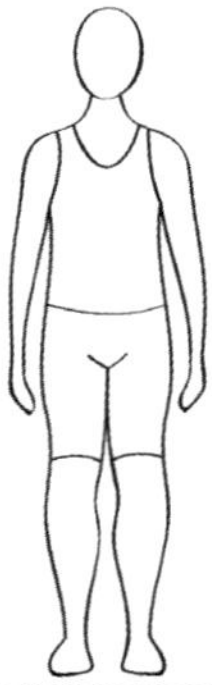

Figure 2.11
Tadasana (Mountain Pose)—roll shoulder up and back five times

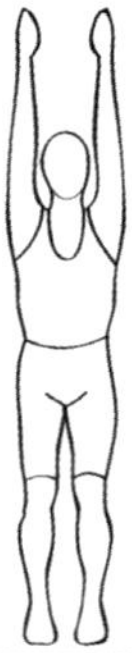

Figure 2.12
Hastasana (Waterfall Pose)

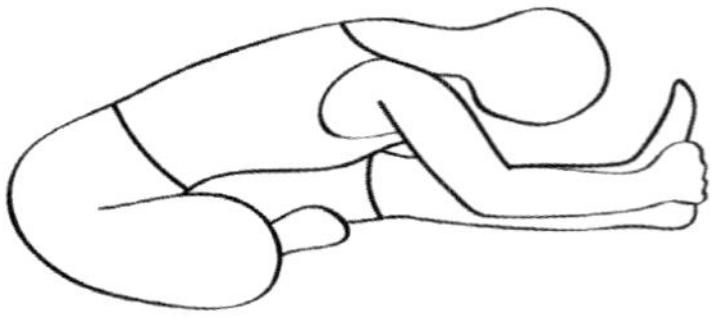

Figure 2.13
Janu Sirsasana (Runner's Stretch)

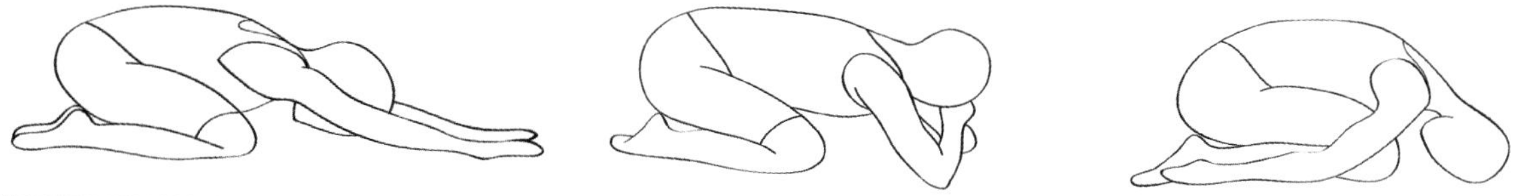

Figures 2.14A, B & C
Pick a variation of Balasana (Child's Pose)

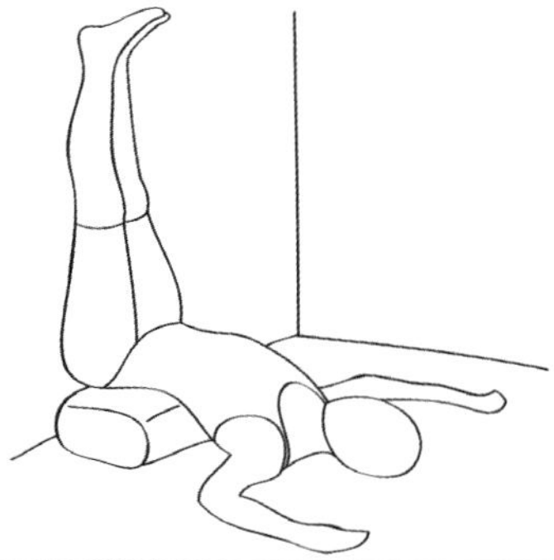

Figure 2.15
Viparita Karani (Legs-up-the-Wall Pose)

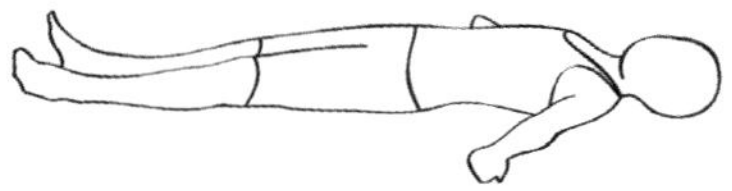

Figure 2.16
Savasana (Relaxation Pose)

C. Adolescents

(Time: 60 minutes)

Working with adolescents is very different from working with either younger children or adults. All their brain structures are operational, like those of an adult, but the brain hasn't been fully myelinated yet as mentioned in Chapter 1. Myelination also increases impulse control, which is part of the reason adolescents may exhibit poor impulse control.

The combination of chronic pain and poor impulse control (due to normal development) can prove to be challenging not only for the adolescent suffering from both, but for the parents and treatment team. A teenage girl who is tired of adhering to treatment guidelines might stop taking an important medication or start engaging in risky behaviors to rebel. Yoga therapy can help teach adolescents the impulse control that they naturally lack. In fact, almost any of the yogic techniques will help with impulse control. However, yoga therapy has to be practiced regularly to be effective. Thus one of the keys to effective yoga therapy for adolescents is helping them determine a routine of yoga practice to maximize its effects. A yoga therapist can do this with the adolescent during the yoga therapy assessment, and then trouble shoot as scheduling problems arise.

As mentioned earlier, chronic pain can lead to anxiety. Unfortunately, deep breathing (which is often used to reduce stress) can sometimes create more anxiety for some Keeping in mind that the purpose of deep breathing for an adolescent with chronic pain is stress relief, I look for alternatives that will have the desired effect. Some effective alternatives for deep breathing include visualizations (such as "Safe Place"), gentle arm movements that mimic the flow of the breath without bringing explicit attention to this, the *Sa Ta Na Ma* mantra, or Child's Pose.

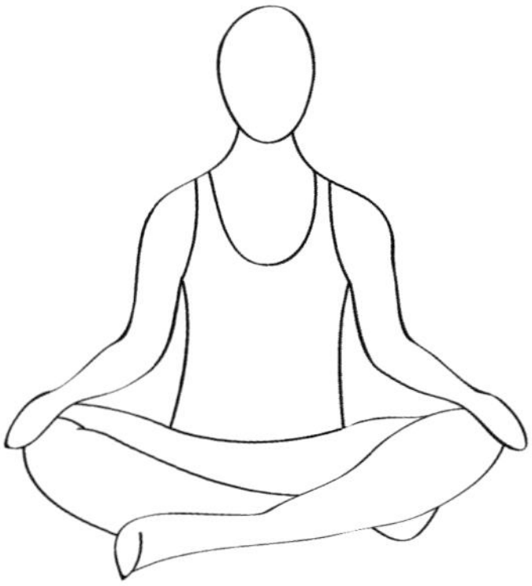

Figure 2.17
Sukhasana (Simple Sitting Pose) with Counting Breaths

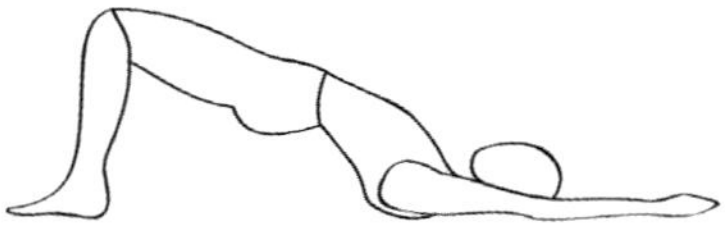

Figure 2.18
Setu Bandha Sarvangasana (Bridge Pose) Vinyasa—repeat five times

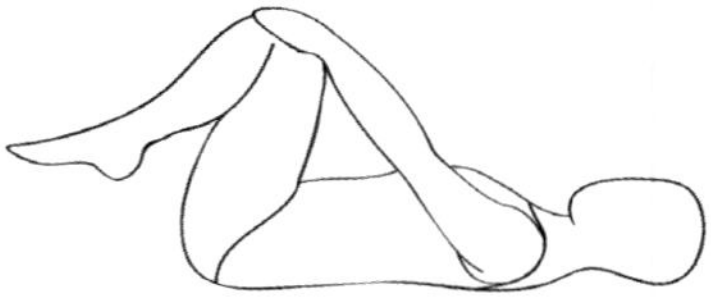

Figure 2.19
Apanasana Vinyasa—repeat 5 – 10 times

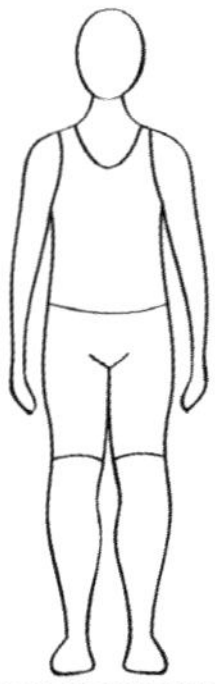

Figure 2.20
Tadasana (Mountain Pose)—roll shoulders up and back five times

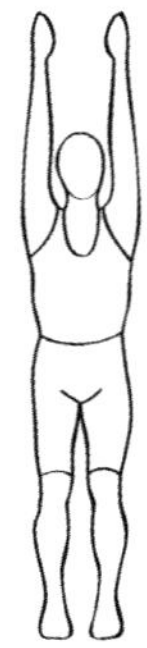

Figure 2.21
Hastasana (Waterfall Pose)

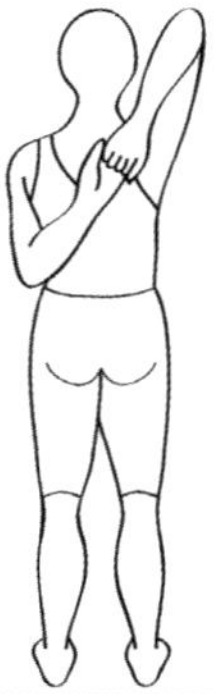

Figure 2.22
Chicken Wing

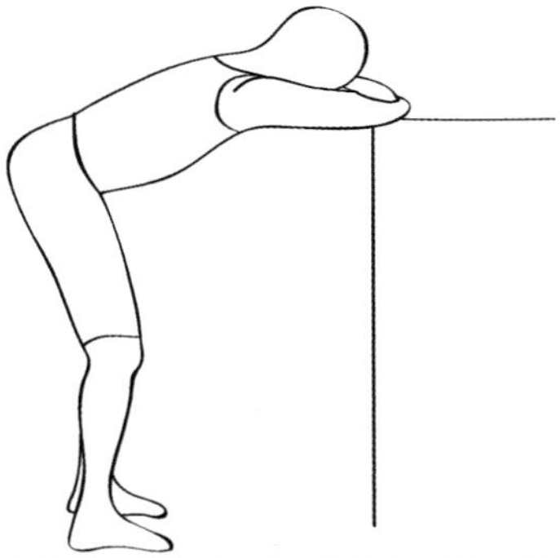

Figure 2.23
Forward fold at table/bar

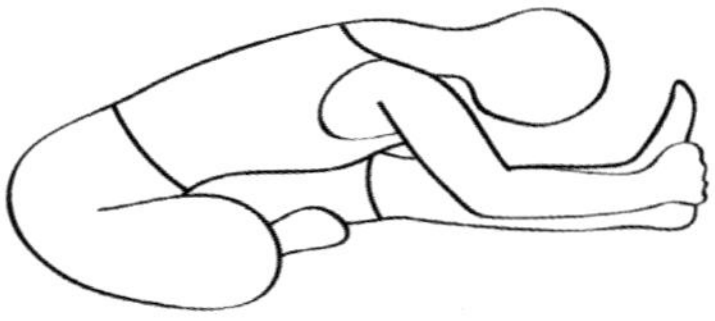

Figure 2.24
Janu Sirsasana (Runner's Stretch)

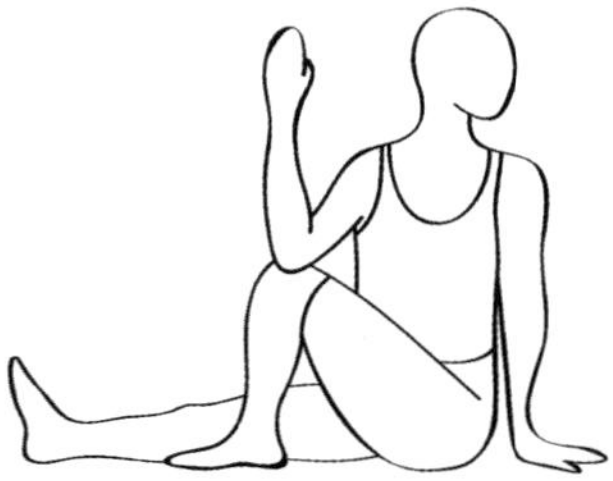

Figure 2.25
Marichyasana C or modification

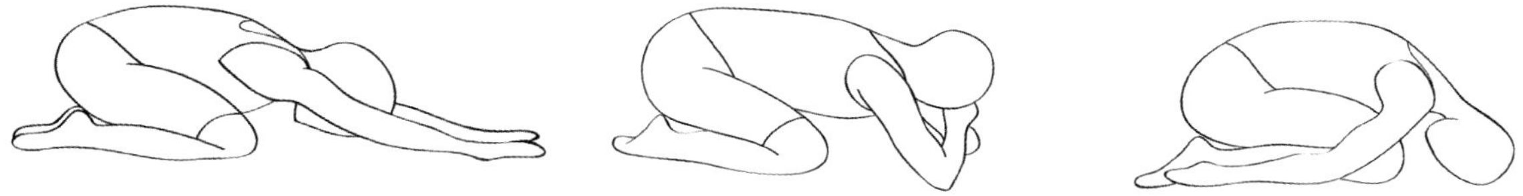

Figures 2.26 A, B & C
Pick a variation of Balasana (Child's Pose)

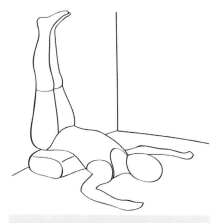

Figure 2.27
Viparita Karani (Legs-up-the-Wall Pose)

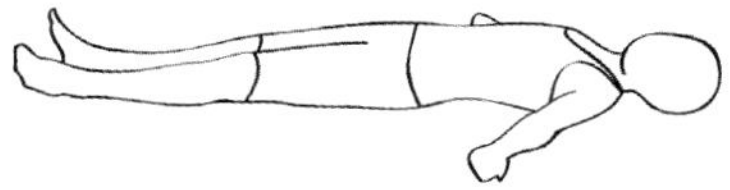

Figure 2.28
Savasana (Relaxation Pose)

Resources

The topic of yoga therapy for chronic pain has received a lot of attention, both in the worlds of allopathic medicine and yoga. As a result, there are a number of yoga sequences available for a variety of pain types. Many of these were originally designed for adults, so I have listed the ones that offer pain management strategies that can be used with youth: Kraftsow (1999) includes a whole chapter on "Common Aches and Pains" in his book *Yoga for Wellness*; McCall (2007) lists several excellent strategies for back ache and chronic headache in *Yoga As Medicine*; and Pearson considers how six of the eight limbs of yoga can be used for general chronic pain in his article "Yoga for People in Pain" in Volume 18 (2008) of *International Journal of Yoga Therapy*. There is also a growing body of work for pediatrics. This includes Evans and colleagues'. (2012) two sequences for rheumatoid arthritis and irritable bowel syndrome, as well as the sequence cited in Hainsworth et al's (2013) article on chronic headache in youth.

Emotion and Behavioral Regulation

3

In samadhi, the last of the eight limbs of yoga, B.K.S. Iyengar says that the "body and senses are at rest . . . (but the) . . . faculties of mind and reason are alert" (1979, p. 52). He says the student becomes both tranquil and alert. Sometimes it is said that samadhi is not actually a yoga practice, but the result of practice. At its heart, samadhi is equilibrium—the ultimate equilibrium, because it cannot be shaken. While the "transcendental state" (Wikipedia, 2014) of samadhi is not the goal of yoga therapy, the goal of any yoga practice is to obtain a sense of equilibrium. Those who struggle with mood dysregulation are constantly buffeted by the emotional ups and downs they experience. Thus, one of the main goals of yoga therapy for mood dysregulation is to restore or gain, perhaps for the first time, some degree of emotional balance and equilibrium.

Mood regulation: An increasingly global concern

The World Health Organization (WHO) released a paper prepared by Kessler and colleagues in 2009 regarding the global burden of "mental disorders." Twenty-eight countries were canvased using the WHO World Mental Health (WMH) survey. Kessler et al. (2009) found that mental health issues are commonly occurring in all participating countries. In particular, two of their findings stand out. The first is that the lifetime prevalence of mental health issues (combining anxiety, mood, externalizing and substance use disorders) worldwide is between 18.1 and 36.1%. The second is the most compelling finding for the purposes of this book, and is that many mental health issues begin in childhood-adolescence. This finding is echoed in the extant literature (Galantino et al., 2008; Birdee et al., 2009; Broderick and Metz, 2009; Greenberg & Harris, 2011). Broderick and Metz (2009) noted that the seeming increase of mental health issues may be due to a greater awareness of mental health issues, as well as increasing stressors on youth.

The WHO report refers to "mental disorders," which connotes formal DSM-5 diagnoses. Diagnostic categories are helpful for specific cases and unique descriptive purposes. However, at the heart of many mental health diagnoses is a problem with emotional and behavioral regulation. In other words, mental health can be seen as one's ability to recognize and manage emotions to an extent that an individual can function without impairment at home, in the community, school, or work settings. As such, I will refer to the difficulty of managing one's mood and emotions as *mood dysregulation*. "Managing" in this context refers to managing or regulating thoughts, feelings and behaviors associated with uncomfortable mood states.

Current research suggests that there is a large degree of overlap among the various anxiety and mood disorders, and that it may be more effective to treat symptomology versus specific diagnoses (Farchione et al., 2012). This treatment approach is called the Transdiagnostic Model, and it "targets negative emotionality and associated psychological difficulties," (Ehrenreich et al., 2009, p. 20). It does this by 1) targeting thoughts leading up to mood dysregulation, 2) reducing and preventing avoidance of dysregulated emotions and 3) encouraging opposite actions to habitual and disordered emotional states. One specific example of a transdiagnostic model is the Unified Protocol. Though the Unified Protocol (UP) was originally developed for adults, Ehrenreich and colleagues adapted it for use in adolescent treatment in a small 2009 study. Yoga therapy fits hand-in-glove with UP's treatment of mood dysregulation. Like UP, yoga discourages avoidance by facilitating present moment awareness of one's total mood state. In addition, yoga by its very nature offers action-oriented strategies for disrupting negative mood states.

In her book *Radical Acceptance* (2003), licensed clinical psychologist and mindfulness teacher Tara Brach says, "By inhabiting my body with awareness, I (discover) the roots of my reactivity" (p. 97). This embodied awareness through yoga teaches self-regulation of emotional states that can provide children and adolescents with an invaluable tool that is theirs for life. Armed with these tools, individuals of any age can self-regulate when inevitable stressors occur in life. Using a mind-body practice like yoga can thereby decrease the likelihood that mental health problems will become serious or entrenched. Practicing yoga can also help reduce the physical sequelae of anxiety and depression (such as migraines, digestive issues and insomnia) (Vadiraja et al., 2009; Wren et al., 2010; Evans et al., 2012; Hainsworth et al., 2013).

Yoga therapy also offers a timely and cost-effective solution for these growing concerns about pediatric mental health (da Silva et al., 2009). This solution is well-timed, given the extent to which mental health problems emerge in childhood and can persist into adulthood across the globe. Yoga is also cost effective, because once learned, it can be practiced on one's own without additional costs like medication, equipment or therapy from a provider.

Supporting evidence

While in its infancy, the evidence to support yoga as an effective tool for pediatric mental health, shows promise for growth and utility. As of February 2014, using three search engines (PubMed, PsychInfo and GoogleScholar), 60 studies were found that explicitly listed yoga and mental health issues in their titles, 59 of which were published in 2004 or later. One study was published in 1990. In nine of the 60 studies, yoga therapy was combined with some other treatment intervention (such as African dance or massage), making it hard to tell how much effect yoga itself had on subjects' mental health. In another eight studies, a mental health diagnosis or concern was listed as secondary to other diagnoses (such as cancer or fibromyalgia).

Two meta-analyses were found, which summarized the research on yoga or yoga therapy for mental health issues (Pilkington et al., 2005; da Silva et al., 2009). Nearly all the studies in the two meta-analyses included adult subjects, most of whom had formal mental health diagnoses. A *meta-analysis* is a study that reviews the existing research on a particular topic. Both meta-analyses looked at whether studies were randomized control trials (RCTs) or not. As mentioned in Chapter 1, an RCT is the "gold standard" of research trials, whereby treatments are rigorously studied to determine their effectiveness. Pilkington and colleagues (2005) evaluated five studies, all of which were RCTs. All subjects in these five studies had a formal diagnosis of depression, ranging from mild to severe. The da Silva et al. (2009) review consisted of 34 studies—17 studies that researched yoga and depression, and 17 studies that researched yoga and anxiety. Fifty-three percent of the depression studies were RCTs, whereas only 35% of the anxiety studies met this research design criteria. Other research methods for either of these groups of studies included open trials, case series or non-randomized. Interestingly, more research has been done on yoga for depression than yoga for anxiety.

The conclusion from the Pilkington and colleagues (2005) meta-analysis was that yoga is potentially beneficial for those suffering from depressive disorders. However, due to issues with methodology in the studies reviewed (such as variation in yoga interventions) the results need to be interpreted with caution. The conclusions from the da Silva et al. (2009) review, which occurred five years later, were that yoga may be comparable to medication, and that the combination of yoga *and* medication is superior to medication alone. In addition, da Silva and colleagues found that yoga may be superior to medication for a subgroup of patients with anxiety, and that yoga may benefit mood and anxiety symptoms associated with medical illness.

The problem remains that these two meta-analyses reviewed studies included adult subjects only. Given the prevalence of mental health issues globally, and its effects on youth (Kessler et al., 2009), it is clear that research needs to be conducted on yoga's efficacy for pediatric mental health, as well as how to translate these results in ways that are meaningful and practical to this demographic. In sum, yoga and/or yoga therapy show great promise as interventions for pediatric depression, anxiety and mood dysregulation, but more rigorous research is required to say conclusively.

Yoga therapy: A timely solution

Yoga shows promise as an effective means for children and adolescents to regulate their moods and emotions—not through didactic learning or simply talking about it, but by feeling it in their bodies and through their emotions (Galantino et al., 2008; Birdee et al., 2009; Broderick & Metz, 2009; Greenberg & Harris, 2011). In my experience, yoga therapy helps young people cultivate emotional balance precisely because it is a mind-body practice. Children and adolescents are encouraged to feel and sense their experience through the yoga postures and techniques, and then learn how to put words to that experience.

Thus, with my experience of leading therapeutic yoga groups, the emerging research in using yoga as a viable treatment for adults, and a need for strategic and prioritized research for the pediatric population, I will outline my conceptualization of how yoga therapy can be used in the treatment of mental health issues for youth.

Conceptualizing yoga therapy for mental health

The research data suggests that yoga helps individuals in three ways:

- it may reduce symptoms of depression (Pilkington et al., 2005; Streeter et al., 2007)
- it may reduce physiological and self-reported symptoms of anxiety (Streeter et al., 2007; Greenberg et al., 2011)
- it is a cost-effective treatment with few, if any, side effects (Pilkington et al., 2005; da Silva et al., 2009).

So how exactly does yoga relieve these symptoms? Or, put another way, how does yoga create emotional balance?

Sutra II.48 of Patanjali's *Yoga Sutras* offers some insight into the second question in particular. It states that yoga *asana* is "accompanied by the relaxation of tension" (Feuerstein, 1989, p. 91). Feuerstein says that what Patanjali is referring to is the "simple psycho-physiological" sensation of the body loosening up. This fits well with my experience as a pediatric yoga therapist: Children and adolescents alike tell me they feel more calm and relaxed after doing yoga. Interestingly, the English pediatrician and psychoanalyst, Donald Winnicott, also linked relaxation in an infant's development to a mind-body experience of feeling safe (1965). He stated that this comes about through "the environmental function of holding" (p. 60).

Holding first happens in the literal sense of a mother holding her child, but later comes to represent an environment that is safe enough for a child to relax (Winnicott, 1965). This is crucial in allowing the baby to develop a healthy sense of self and individuality. "In favorable circumstances the skin becomes the boundary between the me and the not-me. In other words, the psyche has come to live in the soma and an individual's psycho-somatic life has been initiated" (p. 61). This is a key process in human development that not only signals the beginning of a child's awareness of safety in the world but of his own individuality.

Yoga's effectiveness as a mental health therapy may lie in its power to recreate the holding environment for youth, or for any of us for that matter, who didn't experience it as favorably as Winnicott describes. The non-judgmental awareness of present moment experience that one cultivates in yoga, and all mindfulness practices, is similar to this kind of a safe holding environment. Psychiatrist Mark Epstein calls it *bare attention*, which he says affords an individual "a state of unconditional openness that bears an important resemblance to the feeling engendered by an optimally attentive parent" (1995, p. 117). In the research literature, there is agreement that one of the central goals of mindfulness practices like yoga and meditation is a relaxed, open awareness of the present moment with an attitude of acceptance (Pilkington et al., 2005; Greenberg and Harris, 2011), much like bare attention.

However, the bare attention practiced in meditation is a subtle skill that is arguably too subtle for the developing awareness of children and adolescents who experience emotional dysregulation. On the other hand, yoga therapy brings bare attention to a more accessible level of the body. If asked to notice body sensations in the moment even a five year old can identify his heart beating after a rigorous pose, or his shoulders relax after a shoulder stretch. Thus, in pediatric yoga therapy, the child first learns to identify body sensations, and then learns to identify emotions and moods. In this way, pediatric yoga therapy teaches mindfulness of body and emotions in a stepwise process that begins to resemble Epstein's (1995) conception of bare attention, where the individual pays attention to what he is experiencing in the moment, separating emotional reaction from "raw sensory events" (p. 110).

The bare attention that one practices in yoga therapy also cultivates mood and emotion regulation through emotional acceptance. Contrast this to a key feature of emotion and mood dysregulation, known in the field as *emotional avoidance*. Steven Hayes and colleagues (2003) say that emotional avoidance is the unwillingness to recognize thoughts, emotions or bodily sensations arising, as well as an alteration of their "form or frequency" (p. 60). Hayes and colleagues add that "Children are told, regularly and often, that they can and ought to control negative affective states" (p. 62). Yet avoiding emotions habitually can lead to depressive symptoms (p. 61). Thus, cultivating bare attention and emotional acceptance are key components of mental health, and therefore of solid pediatric yoga therapy practice.

Recognizing and accepting emotions

My experience as a yoga therapist working with young people and their families is that practicing bare attention and emotional acceptance happens in three stages: Recognizing emotions, accepting emotions and practicing non-attachment to emotions.

As we have seen from the literature, the problem with emotions is not in having them (Hayes et al., 2003). The problem with emotion and moods is how we *respond* to them (Kabat-Zinn, 1990; Hayes et al., 2003). But first we have to notice our feelings and emotions. Yoga therapy helps children and adolescents slow down enough to notice them. Figure 3.1 illustrates this relationship among normal mood fluctuations versus extreme mood fluctuations into states like major depression or mania.

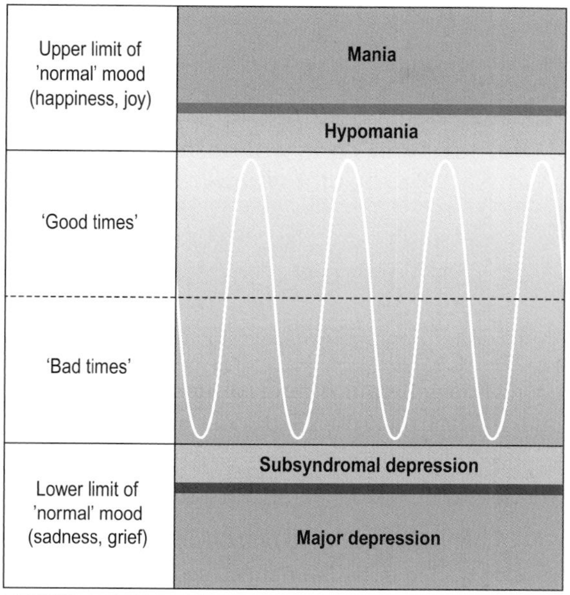

Figure 3.1
The spectrum of mood fluctuations. Reproduced with permission of the Cleveland Clinic Center for Continuing Education. Khalife S, Singh V, Muzina DJ. Bipolar Disorder. Disease Management Project (http://www.clevelandclinicmeded.com/medicalpubs/diseasemanaqement/psvchiatry-psvcholoqy/bipolar-disorder/) ©2000-2011 The Cleveland Clinic Foundation. All rights reserved.

Children (especially pre-schoolers and school-aged children) may not recognize they are having emotions until it is pointed out to them. Or, a child may be so overwhelmed by emotion that she doesn't recognize what she is feeling, or know what to do when feeling uncomfortable or distressed. For instance, I worked with a 12-year-old girl who was admitted to a psychiatric day treatment program for anxiety. She dealt with her anxiety by refusing to go to school, despite having good grades. Most likely, she didn't have any other way to identify or cope with uncomfortable emotions. Her symptoms improved dramatically through intensive and integrated treatment that included yoga therapy. She went back to school, could call friends, and no longer avoided activities that had previously scared her. But she still couldn't identify the feelings that had led to her to refuse school before she started therapy. Interestingly, it appeared she had no problem identifying positive feelings like relaxation or relief in other situations (such as moments in therapy or school when she accomplished a task).

In yoga group, I asked her to pick poses that boosted her confidence, rather than talk about her feelings. She chose Tree, Dancer, Warrior and Crow Poses. During Dancer Pose she casually said before we started the second side, "Oh, this is my bad side."

"Aha!" I said. "That's a worry thought."

"It is?" she and her mother said at the same time.

"Yes, you're worried this side won't be as good as the last," I said.

"Oh, yeah, you're right," she said.

The yoga poses allowed her to notice her worried, anxious thoughts in an activity she likes (yoga) without the usual panic and self-esteem issues that came up for her at school. In essence, yoga sessions became a safe "holding environment" (Winnicott, 1965). Because she felt safe in yoga, she was willing to take more risks by doing challenging yoga poses that she sometimes fell out of. Also, because she felt safe she was willing to try again and use coping thoughts like, "I can do this!" By the end of her treatment she could identify her feelings of anxiety and panic in school and social situations. She even helped explain how to identify feelings to a new participant two weeks later, a relational skill called *mirroring* (Winnicott, 1971).

Once a child recognizes what he feels, the next step is accepting it. "Psychologically, (emotional acceptance) connotes an active taking in of an event or situation" (Hayes et al., 2003, p. 77). Accepting emotions as they are can seem counterintuitive to children and adolescents (and their families) who are being seen for behavioral problems related to their emotions, such as angry outbursts or suicidal thoughts. Yoga therapy helps an individual recognize emotions and then pause before acting, or reacting as the case may be. This slowing down process is what allows the individual to see that accepting one's emotions allows one to respond rather than react to those emotions. In fact, changing a behavior related to emotion dysregulation requires that the individual first recognize and accept the disturbing emotion or mood that prompts the dysfunctional behavior.

For example, one adolescent I worked with was admitted for anxiety and depression. One of his main fears was that he would be shot at school. Unfortunately in the United States, this is not an irrational fear, given the number of school shootings we have seen in the last 20 years. This young man had a natural emotional response to an unnaturally stressful life circumstance.

In his case, this adolescent's emotional response overruled his ability to engage in the activities that gave his life meaning, such as going to school and hanging out with friends. During the few times I saw him in yoga group, he was able to use deep breathing to slow down his perseverating thoughts and simply watch his breath. After deep breathing one morning, he had the insight that going to school and successfully graduating were important steps toward his future career, whatever that might be. He was able to slow down and identify uncomfortable feelings of panic about going back to school. Not only that, he was able to identify the feelings of panic without reacting to them—the essence of emotional acceptance. In this way, he was able to integrate what he had learned and state an important insight during this particular session.

Non-attachment to emotions

Once a child can recognize and accept his emotion, he then has the power to remain calm in the face of emotional states that may have led him to unhealthy behaviors in the past. In yoga therapy this point is pivotal, and is best stated in the oft-quoted second aphorism (sutra I.2) of Patanjali's Yoga Sutras: *yogas citta vrtti nirodhah.* Prabhavananda and Isherwood (1981) translate it as, "Yoga is the control of thought waves in the mind" (p. 15). Here we could easily replace the word "thought" with "emotion."

Medical doctor and mindfulness pioneer Jon Kabat-Zinn, M.D., often refers to emotions as waves and emotional states as weather patterns (1990). In his ground-breaking book, *Full Catastrophe Living* (1990), he uses the term "non-attachment" in relation to emotional states to describe the process of recognizing that emotions are temporary states – not the essence of who we are.

In learning non-attachment to emotions, the individual first engages in "an active process of feeling feelings as feelings" (Hayes et al., 2003, p. 77), another way of viewing emotional acceptance. By viewing feelings as feelings, the individual naturally creates some distance from them. Feelings come and go. By not being so caught up in them, an individual has more choice about how to act. The same teen I mentioned above was able to detach from his feelings of panic and despair to see the bright future he wanted. He did this by breathing deeply, which he said slowed down his thinking and allowed him to notice his emotions changing. The change he reported was that he felt calmer. He had to recognize and accept his anxiety and depression before he could detach from it.

Current evidence-based treatments like Cognitive Behavioral Therapy (CBT) and Dialectical Behavioral Therapy (DBT) use slowing down as a means to improved emotion regulation, much like yoga therapy. However, I believe the difference with yoga therapy is that it includes the body more explicitly and directly. The child practices slowing down in an integrated, mind-body approach. To further highlight how yoga therapy helps youth cultivate slowing the mind and body down through recognizing emotions, accepting emotions and practicing non-attachment, two case study composites follow.

Case studies

Jessica

"Jessica" is a 15-year-old girl, who was hospitalized for severe stomach pains that were diagnosed as stomach migraines (a clinical diagnosis for extreme stomach pain with symptoms similar to migraine headaches), and associated weight loss. While Jessica was in the hospital, she was referred to me to help her manage panic attacks and stomach pain. I taught her how to slow down her breathing, and then lengthen her exhalation. She reported that lengthening her exhalation calmed her down and reduced her pain. Several months after she was discharged from the hospital, she began having panic attacks again and couldn't maintain a healthy body weight as she entered her freshman year of high school. When Jessica had a panic attack, she became short of breath and felt a feeling of dread. Her stomach migraines caused her such pain that she had to be admitted to the hospital again. Her mother reminded her how much she benefited from deep breathing, and so I began to see her in our outpatient clinic once a week for several months.

Jessica's physical and emotional symptoms clearly indicated anxiety as the primary issue. Jessica's stomach migraines worsened with stress in her life, as did her panic attacks. Someone who experiences anxiety like Jessica needs a chance to diffuse her pent-up energy before slowing down. Of course, Jessica is not alone in her need for this approach. Many of us who experience stress and anxiety also need to release tension before relaxation is possible. As such, often Jessica and I spent the first half of the session practicing sun salutations and active poses. Once she felt relaxed enough she could sit and practice deep breathing, after which we would talk to debrief her feelings and progress in the session. She said that the vigorous sun salutations helped her manage her anxiety and reflect on her life. Over the course of our work together, she was able to channel her high energy into things she loved like basketball and being a leader in different clubs at school.

Aidan

In Chapter 1, I introduced "Aidan," a 13-year-old male whose behavior is consistent with Bipolar II Disorder. Whereas Jessica mostly struggled with the frantic energy of anxiety, Aidan's moods regularly swing from depressed and irritable to manic and violent . In the following narrative, I reintroduce Aidan to contrast his yoga therapy program with Jessica's. To empower Aidan and respect his developmental need for choice and autonomy, I told Aidan he was in charge: He was responsible for telling me how much energy he had at the beginning of the session, and whether he needed to increase or decrease that energy. He became skilled at naming his own state and deciding what yoga techniques would help If he was feeling manic, we would start our session with some high energy poses until, like Jessica, he was able to slow down to calmer techniques like deep breathing. When he reported low energy at the beginning of a session, not only would we do gentler practices

Case studies *(Continued)*

at the beginning, but I would also use more step-by-step verbal cues to help structure his experience and maintain his focus for longer. My added cuing helped keep him focused and moving, versus giving in to his depressed state.

In summary

In this chapter we have explored the emerging research regarding the application of yoga for mental health, almost all of which used adult subjects. Clearly, there is a need for well-designed research in pediatric yoga therapy, given the growing worldwide concern of mental health issues like depression (Kessler et al., 2009). In a sense, this chapter is a call to arms to researchers, pediatric providers and yoga therapists alike to collaboratively create yogic interventions that are systemized, and can be replicated, so that we may research their benefit for children and adolescents.

The first step in systemizing yoga interventions for mood regulation is to clarify our approach to mental health in youth. Rather than focus on diagnoses, a new transdiagnostic model called the Unified Protocol focuses on symptoms (Farchione et al., 2012). This is a more balanced and appropriate approach to exploring mental well-being in children and adolescents, whose behaviors and tendencies change as they grow and mature. Pediatric yoga therapy can be a great adjunctive treatment to this approach by offering individualized care that considers the whole child (mind and body) to optimize her mental well-being.

Another important aspect of systemizing pediatric yoga therapy is integrating care. When a yoga therapist collaborates with a child's clinical team, including parents or other caregivers, mental health provider(s), medical doctor, and/or important teachers, the child and the whole team benefit from a more complete view of the child's strengths and needs. The yoga therapist works with this team to create a yoga therapy program that facilitates:

1 recognizing emotions
2 accepting emotions
3 non-attachment to emotional states.

A child's ability to master these steps depends a lot on his current level of development. In addition, because anxiety and depression often go hand in hand, a yoga therapist must be sensitive to what state a child or adolescent is currently in when prescribing practice for mood regulation. Yoga therapy for mood regulation is not a one-size-fits-all endeavor. For instance, adolescents with anxious affect generally do better with a high-energy practice that progresses to slower, calmer movements and techniques. Adolescents with depressed affect do well with a gentle beginnings that progress to more active poses, such as standing poses and backbends. They also benefit from more frequent cueing from the yoga therapist to keep their minds busy and distracted from negative thoughts.

Finally, yoga therapy offers a cost-effective solution for growing concerns about pediatric mental health (Pilkington et al., 2005; da Silva et al., 2009). Yoga is a mind-body practice that increases awareness of one's inner world, and this teaches self-regulation of emotional states that can provide children and adolescents with an invaluable tool they possess for the rest of their lives.

Practice considerations

When it comes to designing a yoga therapy intervention for youth struggling with mood regulation, behavioral profile is just as important as age. For instance, in a group of 10 teens, three teens may be severely depressed and struggling with suicidal ideation, three teens experiencing hallucinations, and the other four rapidly cycling from anxiety to depression (e.g. bipolar mood swings). The job of a yoga therapist is to design a yoga intervention that helps the entire group regulate their moods, or learn to be present with uncomfortable thoughts, feelings and sensations. These two factors of age and behavioral profile help one determine the length of time of the yoga session, as well as the number and type of yogic practices to be used. Refer to Chapter 1 for time and instruction guidelines for the different age groups. With regards to behavioral profile, more specific guidelines are offered below.

Another important consideration is: what other professionals are working with the child and family? Depending on the setting, this team may be a formal treatment team gathered in one organization, but more likely it will be a collection of community providers. It is best practice for the yoga therapist to first obtain consent from the child and guardian(s), and then to discuss the case with the other treating clinicians or providers. In this way, the yoga therapist can create an integrated assessment of the child's needs that informs the yoga therapy treatment plan. The treatment team includes the child, the parents (or other family or caregivers), and possibly a primary psychologist or psychotherapist, psychiatrist, social worker, medical doctor, and/or important teacher(s).

Practices for mood regulation

Pre-schoolers

As mentioned previously, the main objective for this age group is to have fun, and learn a little about self-regulation practices. A yoga therapist should not expect to lead the sample practice in the exact order listed below. Children at this age need the freedom to play and explore. So it's best to come up with a broad theme like "animals," and find ways to incorporate mental balance within the theme. For instance, if a group of children enjoys practicing Snake Breath, the yoga therapist can suggest having a contest to see who can hiss the longest. (Forewarning: Don't introduce breathing exercises that require counting, as many children of this age can't count very far yet.) Refer to Chapter 9 for detailed instructions, modifications and contraindications of the poses.

Ring a bell to indicate the beginning of the yoga therapy session.

School-aged children

For school-aged children, using yoga to identify and accept emotions may be an entirely nonverbal practice. For instance, making vocalizations of a happy and angry cat in Cat-Cow Pose can teach a child how to play-act emotions. When the spine is extended and the head looking up, the yoga therapist cues the child to make "happy cat" sounds. And when the spine is in flexion and the child is looking at his belly button, the yoga therapist cues the child to make "angry cat" sounds. The permission to act out an angry cat can be so freeing that everyone—children, yoga therapist, and any onlookers—find themselves having a good laugh. This is a good stage to intro-

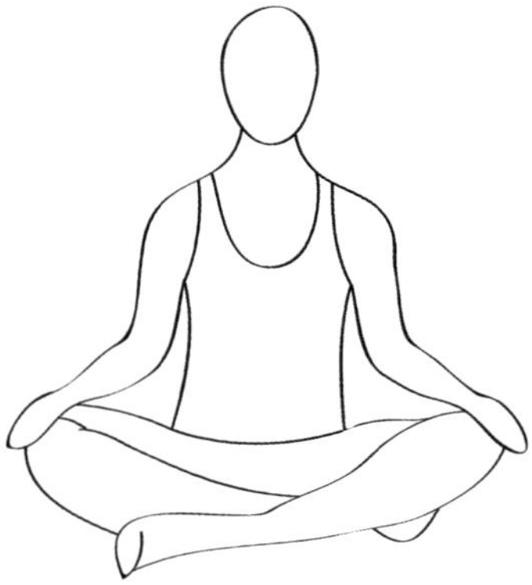

Figure 3.2
Sukhasana (Simple Sitting Pose) with Snake Breath

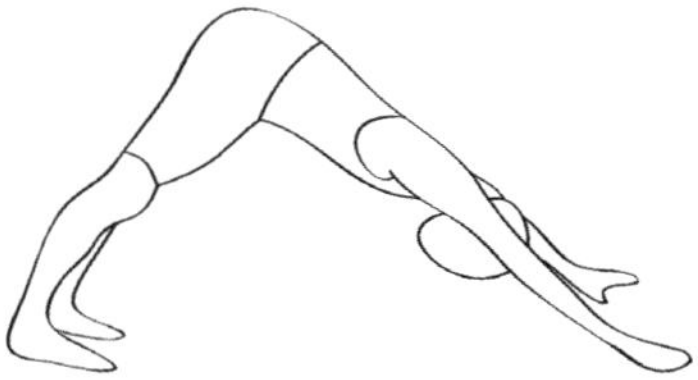

Figure 3.3
Adho Mukha Svanasana (Downward-facing Dog)

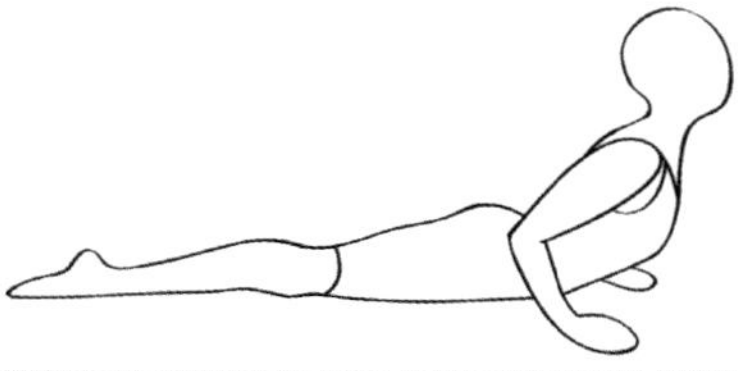

Figure 3.4
Bhujangasana (Cobra Pose)

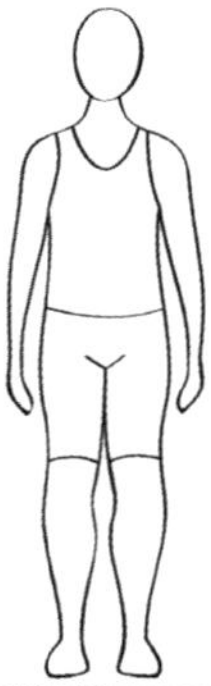

Figure 3.5
Tadasana (Mountain Pose)

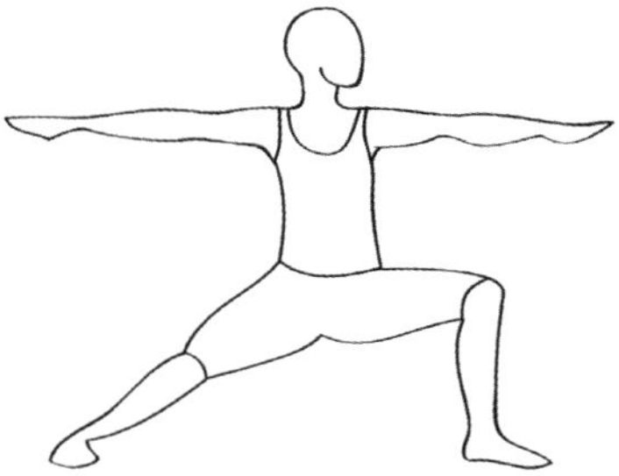

Figure 3.6
Virabhadrasana II (Warrior II)

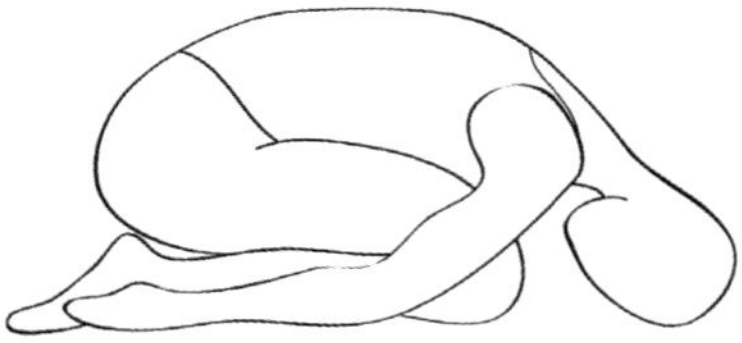

Figure 3.7
Balasana (Child's Pose)

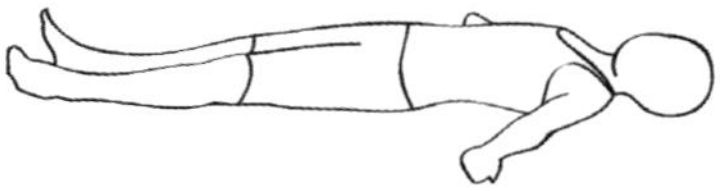

Figure 3.8
Savasana with beanie baby, or other soft, weighted object, on belly to feel breathing

duce concentration as a way to regulate mood. One of the most effective tools I have found is ringing a bell that reverberates for a while. Instruct the children to close their eyes to reduce other distractions and then raise their hands the first second they no longer hear sound from the bell.

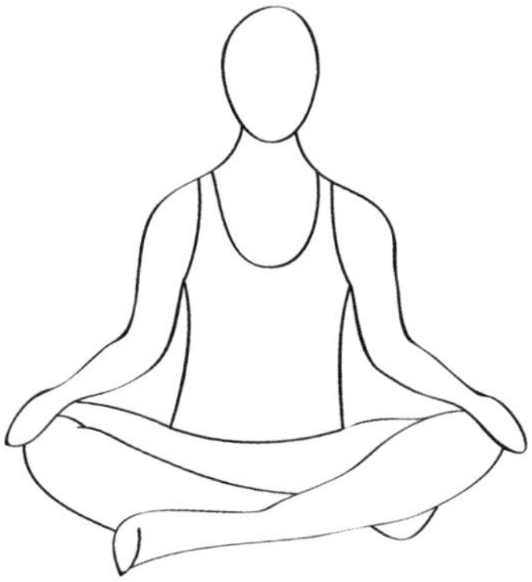

Figure 3.9
Sukhasana (Simple Sitting Pose) with Snake Breath

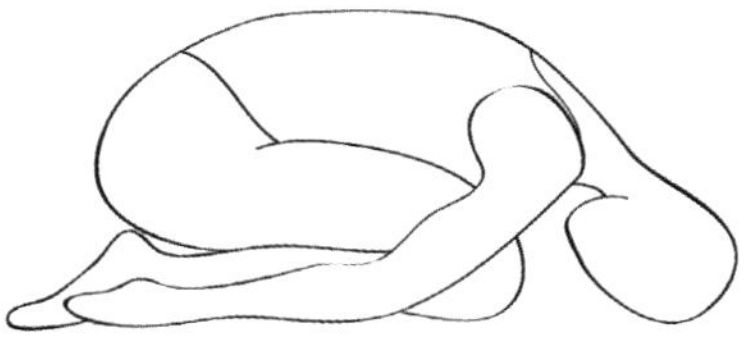

Figure 3.10
Balasana (Child's Pose)

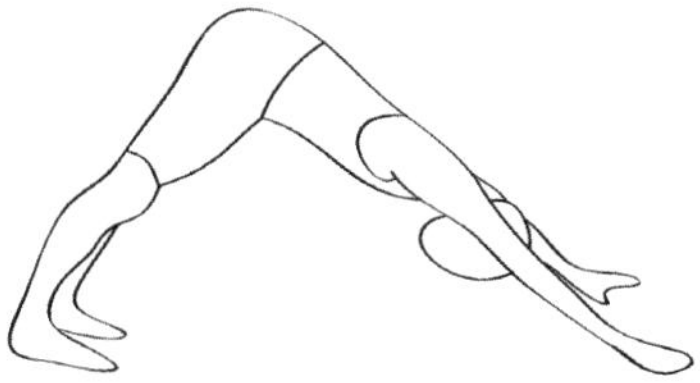

Figure 3.11
Adho Mukha Svanasana (Downward-facing Dog)

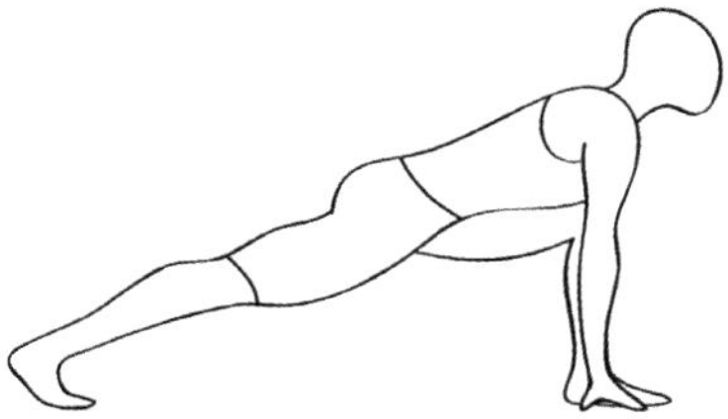

Figure 3.12
Lunge—repeat on both sides

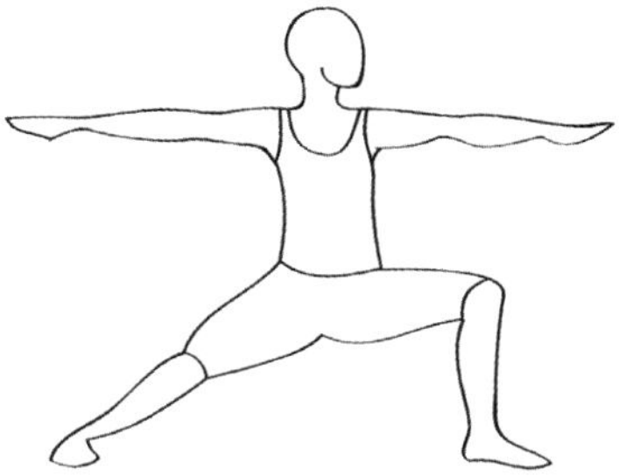

Figure 3.13
Virabhadrasana II (Warrior II)—repeat on both sides

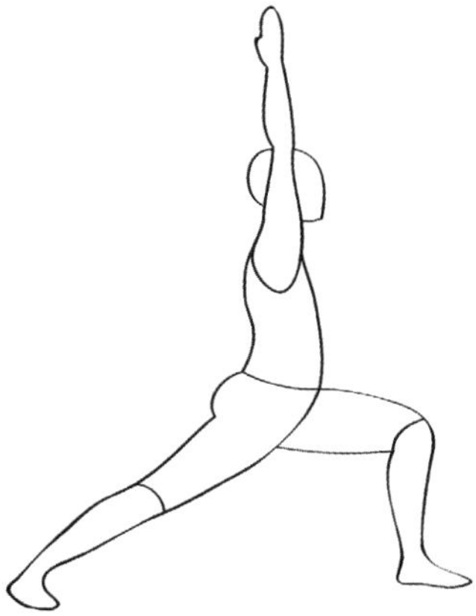

Figure 3.14
Virabhadrasana I (Warrior I)—repeat on both sides

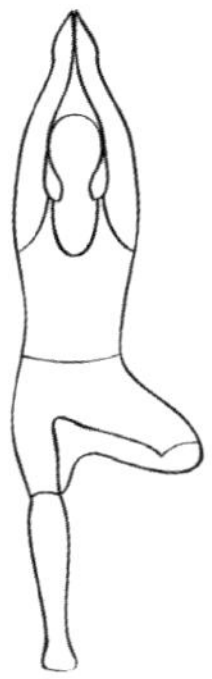

Figure 3.15
Vrksasana (Tree Pose)—repeat on both sides

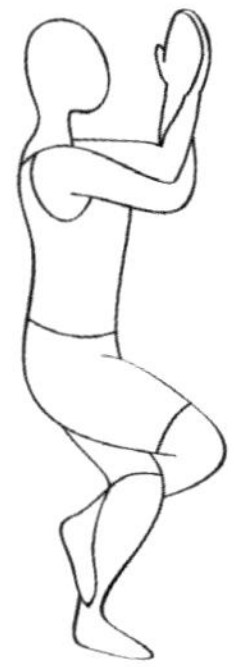

Figure 3.16
Garudasana (Eagle Pose)—repeat on both sides

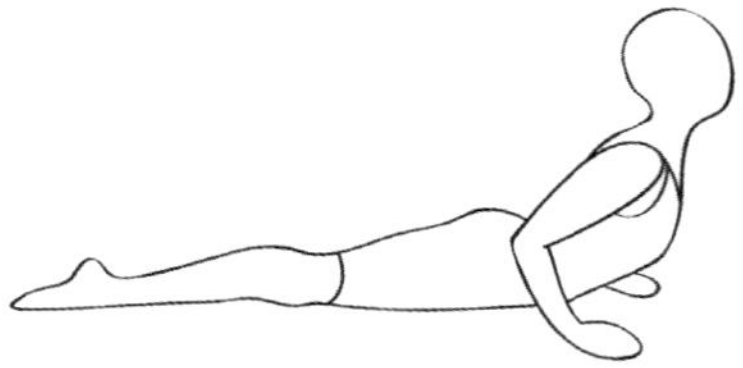

Figure 3.17
Bhujangasana (Cobra)

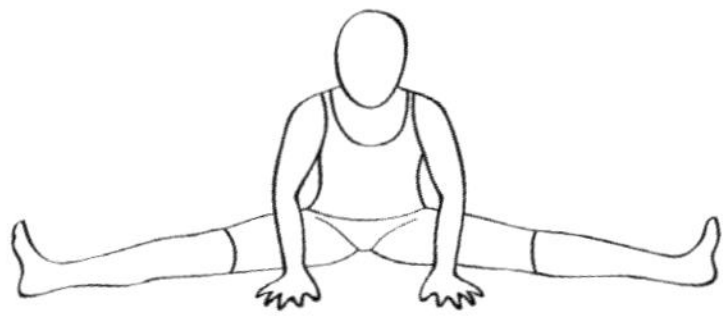

Figure 3.18
Upavistha Konasana (Seated Wide-Angle Pose)

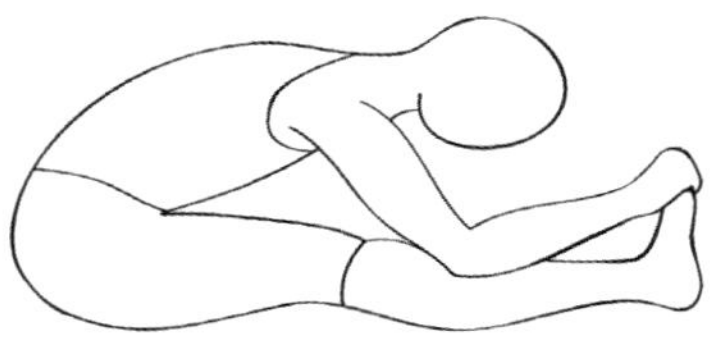

Figure 3.19
Paschimottanasana (Seated Forward Fold)

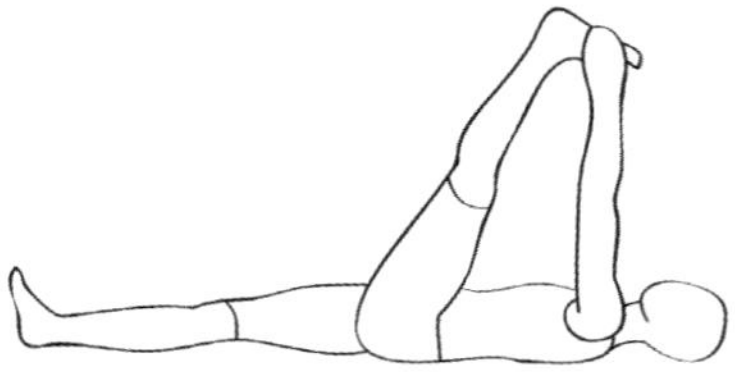

Figure 3.20
Supta Padangusthasana (Supine Leg Stretch)

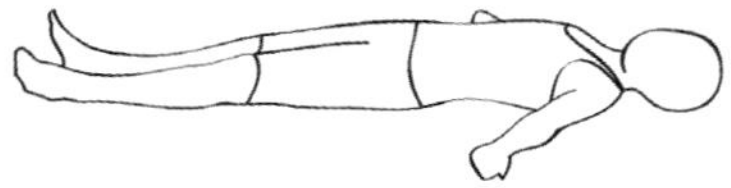

Figure 3.21
Savasana with Five-Minute Vacation Relaxation

Adolescents

Often, I will start practice with a whimsical "ice-breaker" question like, "If you had an empty pool what would you fill it with?" I also make sure to ask about injuries, given that many adolescents are involved in team sports. Meanwhile, I take note of the nonverbal cues: eye contact, body posture, and facial expressions to determine the dominant emotions of the group. Then I guide the adolescent group through a slow flow of yoga poses to help me assess their mobility, strength and stamina.

Most adolescents love standing balances like Tree and Airplane Poses. Back-bending and standing yoga poses are good for adolescents with depressed affect (Shapiro & Cline, 2004; Woolery et al., 2004). More athletic ado lescents who present with anxious affect often benefit from more challenging arm balances like Crow Pose or Handstand at the Wall. Whereas the two younger age-group practices focused on overall mental balance, I have included two different practices for adolescents to further illustrate the case studies in this chapter—one for primary anxious symptoms and one for primary depressive symptoms.

Practice for adolescents with symptoms of anxiety

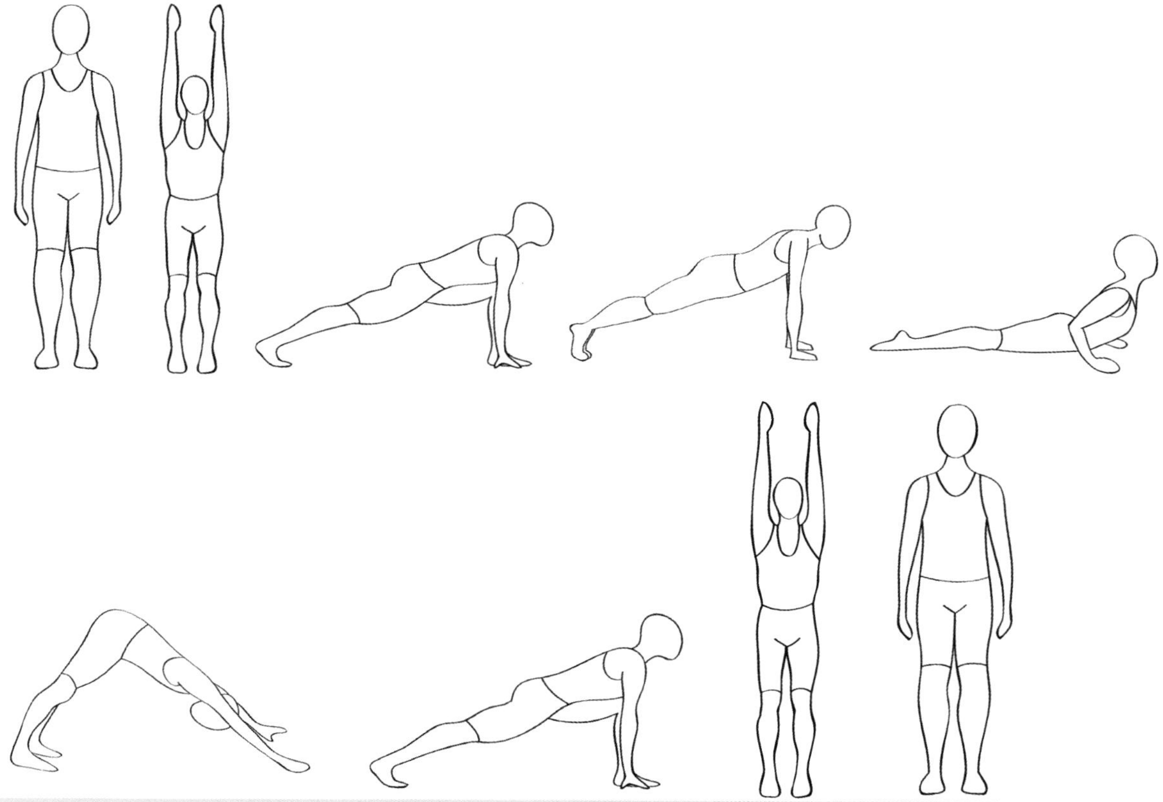

Figure 3.22
Surya Namaskar (Sun Salutation)—repeat this vinyasa three times

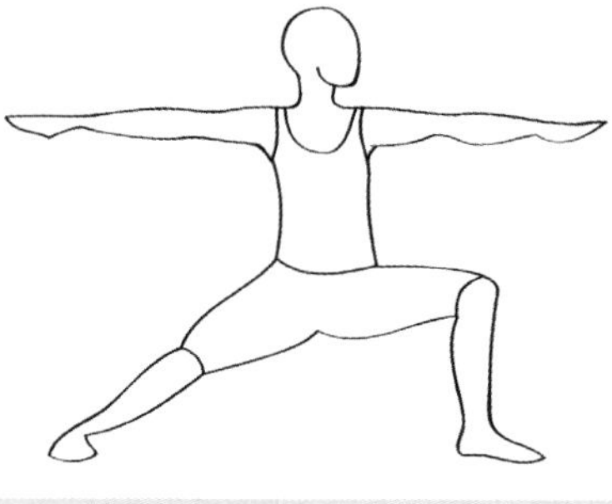

Figure 3.23
Virabhadrasana II (Warrior II)—
repeat on both sides

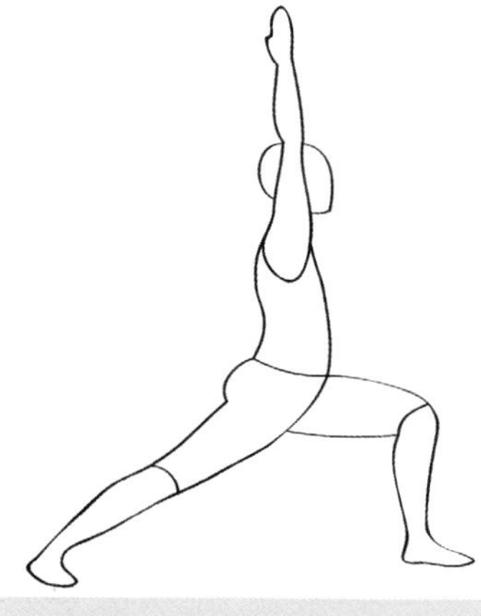

Figure 3.24
Virabhadrasana I (Warrior I)—
repeat on both sides

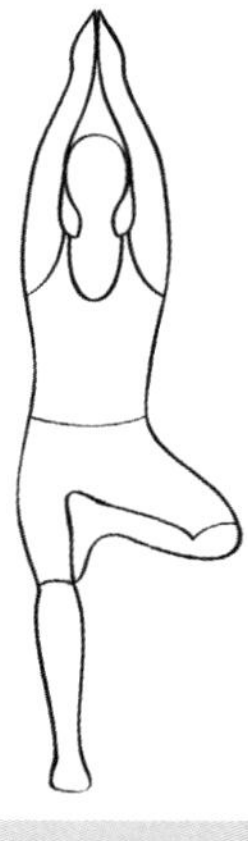

Figure 3.25
Vrksasana (Tree Pose)—repeat on
both sides

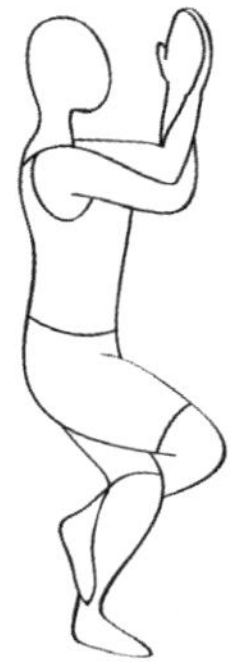

Figure 3.26
Garudasana (Eagle Pose)—repeat on both sides

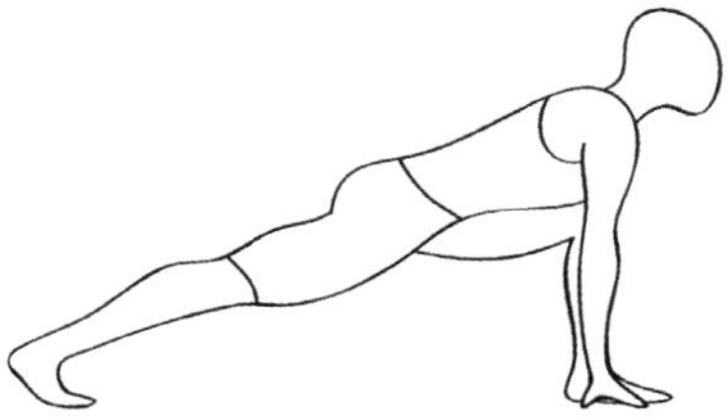

Figure 3.27
Lunge—repeat on both sides

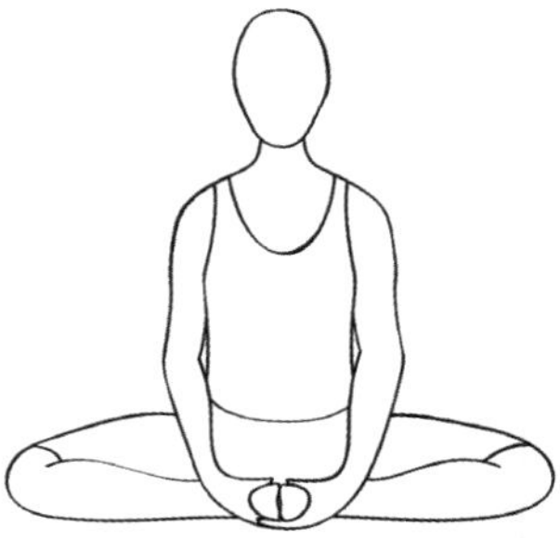

Figure 3.28
Baddha Konasana A or B

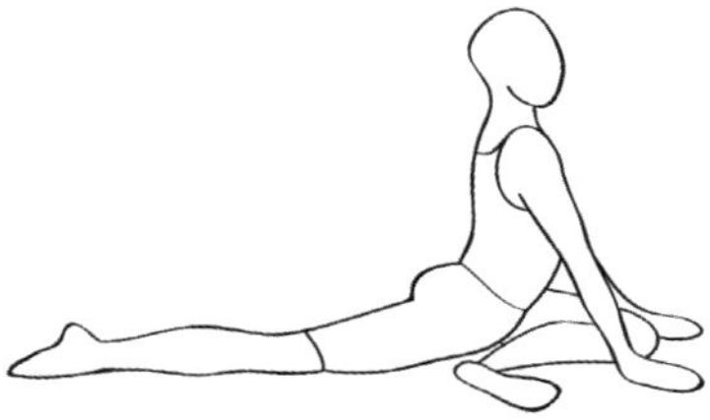

Figure 3.29
Eka Pada Rajakapotasana prep (Pigeon Pose)—repeat on both sides

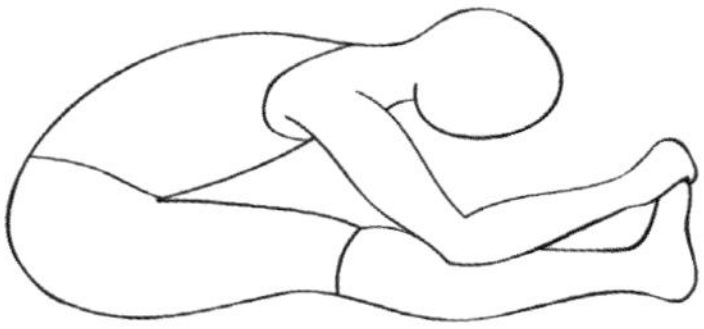

Figure 3.30
Paschimottanasana (Seated Forward Fold)

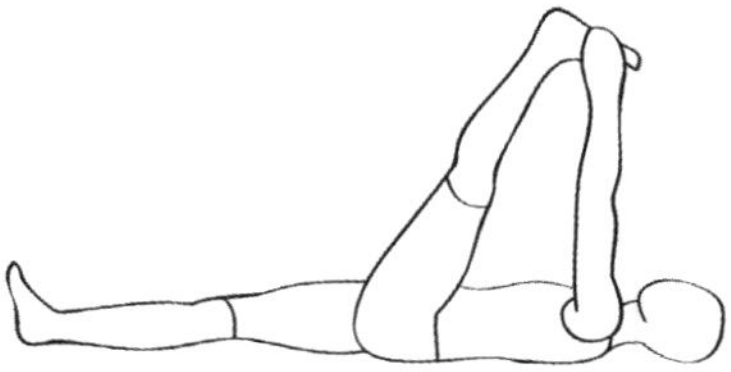

Figure 3.31
Supta Padangusthasana (Supine Leg Stretch)

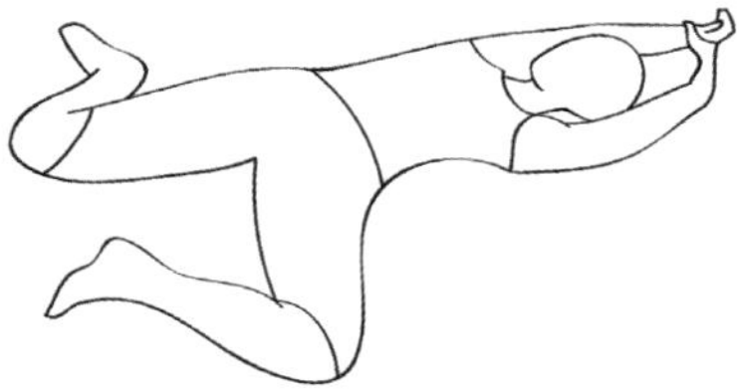

Figure 3.32
Windshield wipers

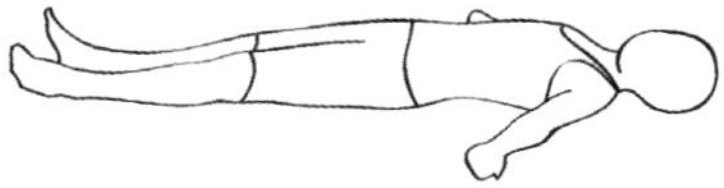

Figure 3.33
Savasana with short Yoga Nidra (5–10 minutes)

Practice for adolescents with symptoms of depression

If an individual is experiencing severe symptoms of depression, the sun salutation may not feel possible. In this case, replace the sun salutation with a standing pose or two, or another pose with which the individual feels more comfortable. The deeper backbend at the end of the practice (*Purvottanasana*) can also be omitted. It is better to do a slower or less physically engaging practice than none at all.

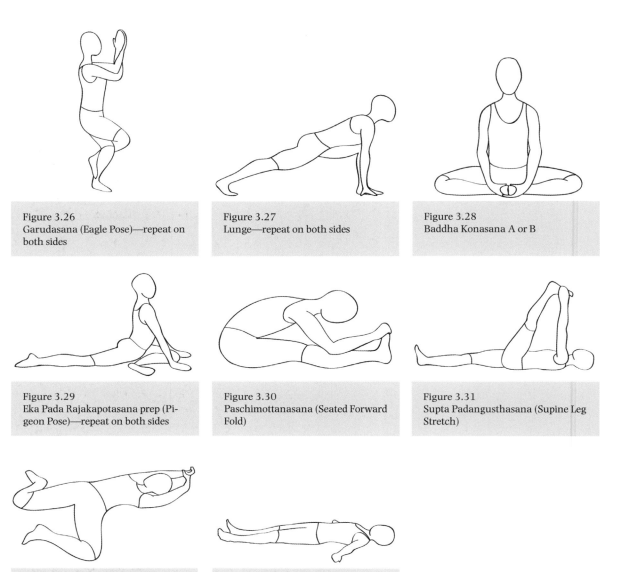

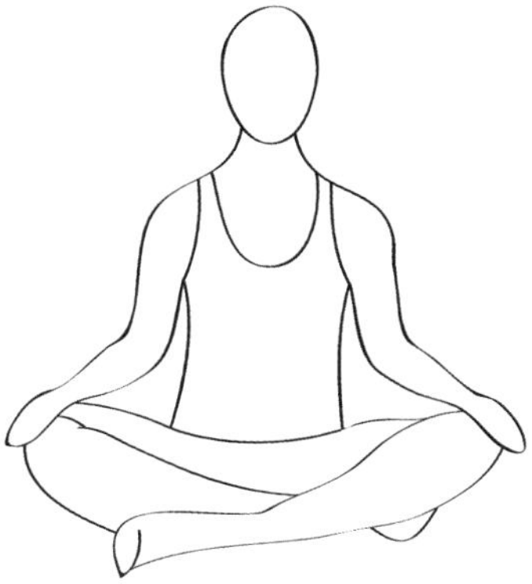

Figure 3.34
Sukhasana (Simple Sitting Pose) with arm raises (3–5 times) and deep breathing

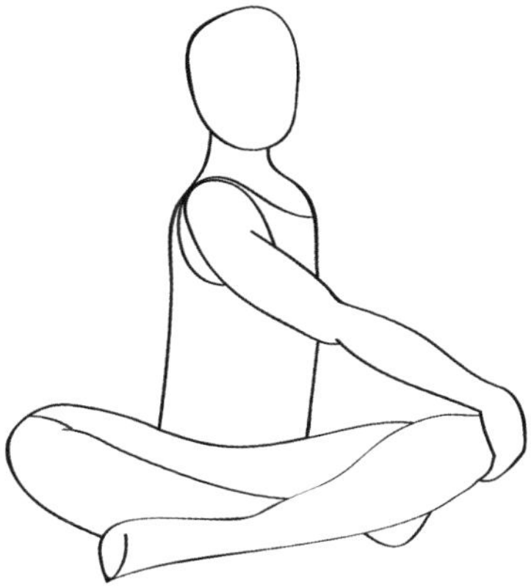

Figure 3.35
Sukhasana Twist (Seated Twist)—repeat on both sides

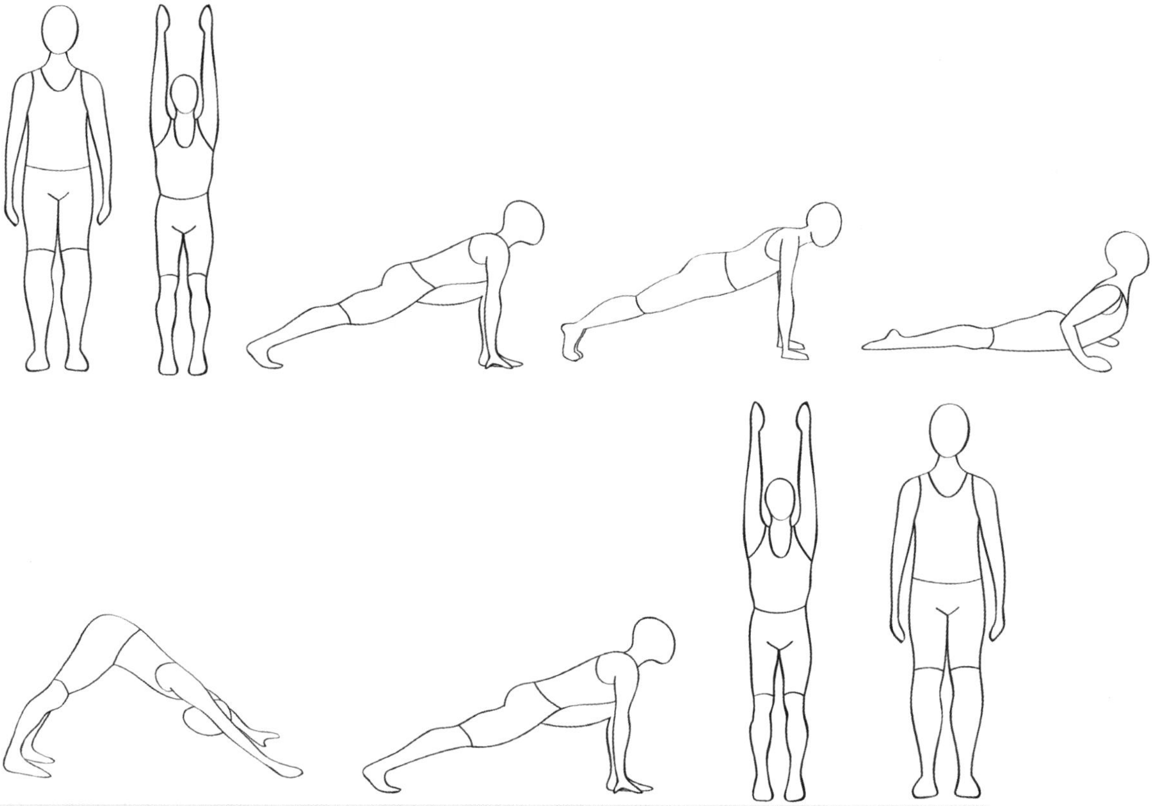

Figure 3.36
Surya Namaskar (Sun Salutation)—repeat this vinyasa three times

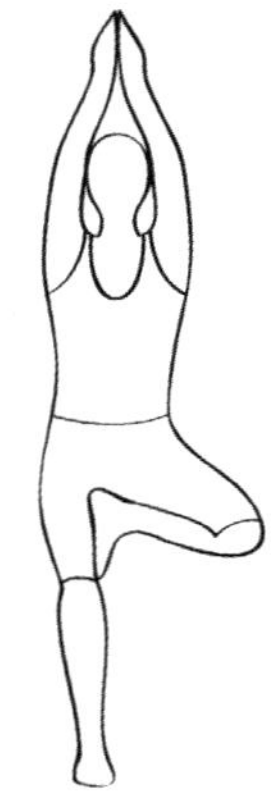

Figure 3.37
Vrksasana (Tree Pose)

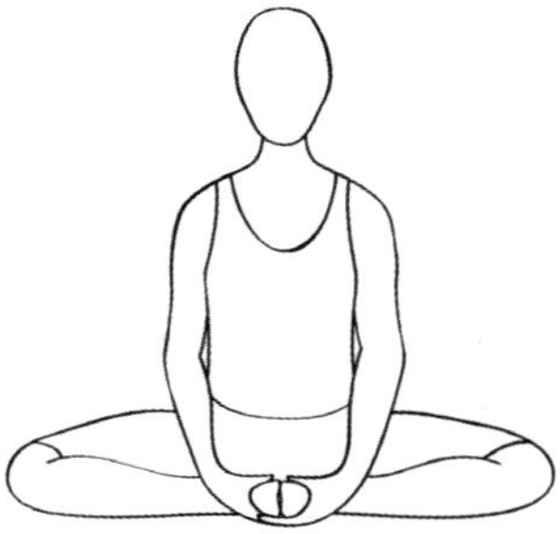

Figure 3.38
Baddha Konasana A (Cobbler's Pose)

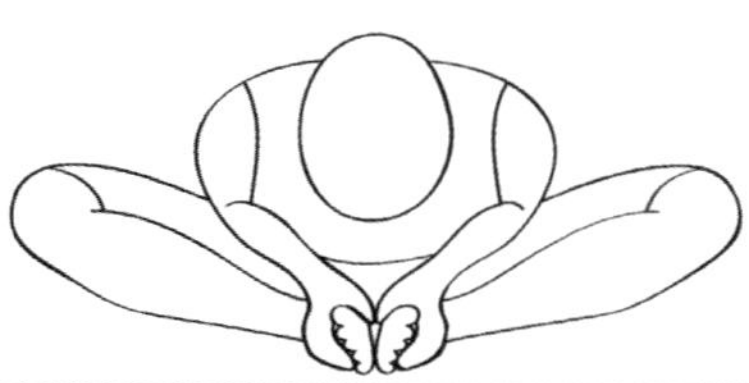

Figure 3.39
Baddha Konasana B (Cobbler's Pose B)

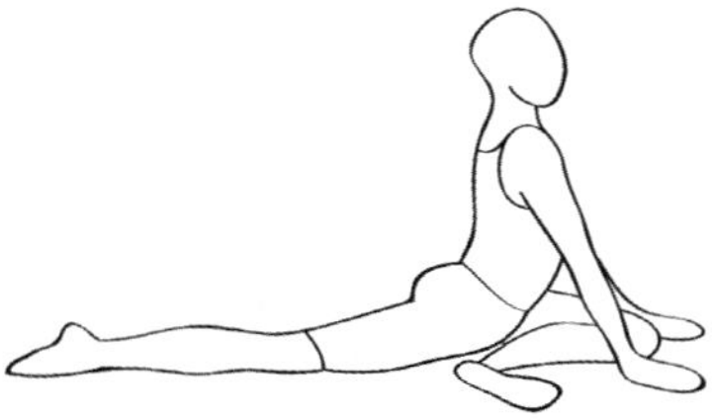

Figure 3.40
Eka Pada Rajakapotasana prep (Pigeon Pose)—repeat on both sides

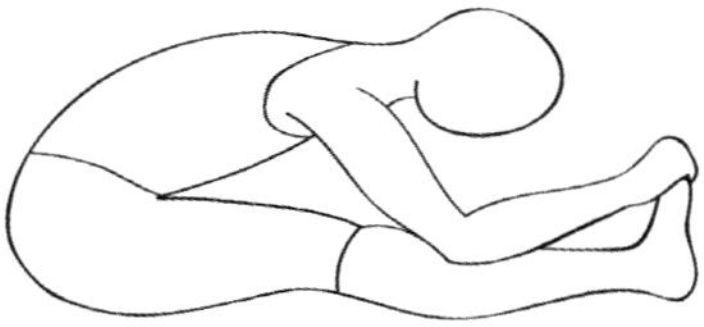

Figure 3.41
Paschimottanasana (Seated Forward Fold)

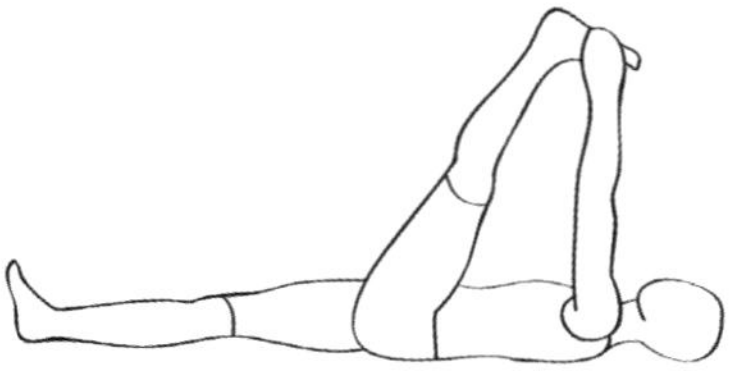

Figure 3.42
Setu Bandha Sarvangasana (Bridge Pose) Vinyasa—repeat five times

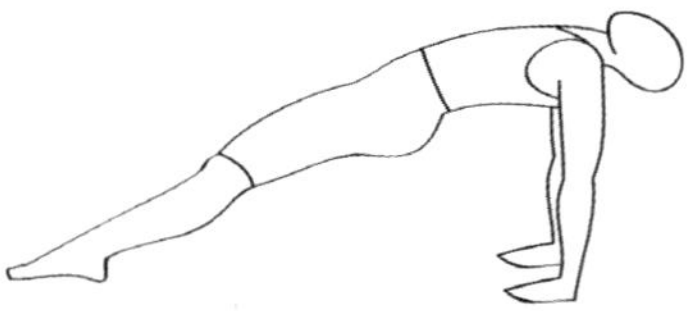

Figure 3.43
Purvottanasana (Upward Plank Pose)

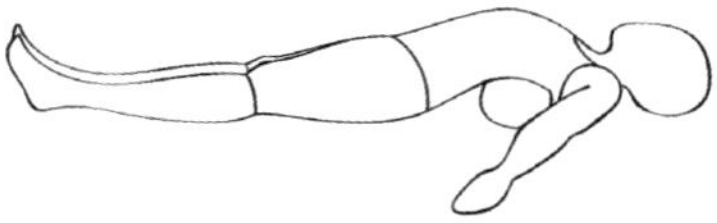

Figure 3.44
Supported Backbend

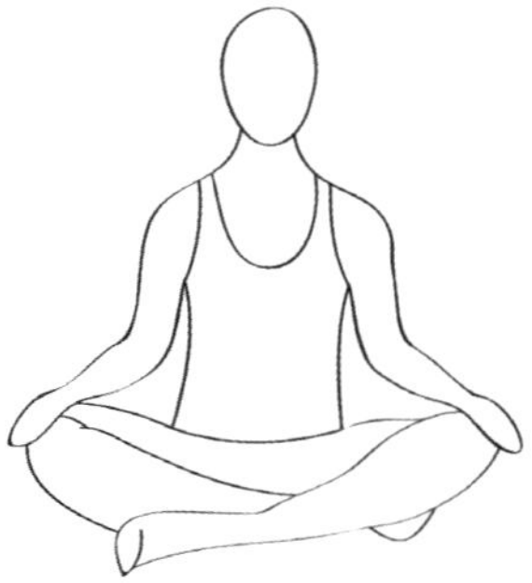

Figure 3.45
Sitting in Sukhasana, practice Sa Ta Na Ma mantra described on pp 110-111 instead of Savasana.

Yoga Therapy for Symptoms of Trauma

4

Trauma, the Space Invader; "Where do you feel that in your body?" I asked.

"I ... I don't know," my client said. "It's like I don't even exist anymore. There's just this . . . this feeling of panic, terror."

I was an intern therapist at the local rape crisis center, and was asking my 18-year-old client to describe where she felt the panic and terror. Yet she couldn't describe what the terror felt like, or locate it in her body. I knew that her lack of bodily awareness (despite her reports that the feelings were overwhelming) was normal for someone who has experienced a trauma. "How big is the terror and panic?" I asked.

"Uh, well it's everywhere. It's hard to describe where it's not*, so I'm not sure how big it is."*

"Wow, that sounds huge," I said. Still a therapist-in-training, I remembered something my internship supervisor had said about ACT (Acceptance and Commitment Therapy). She had told me that ACT therapists use outrageous scenarios with clients in order to help them see their situation in a new light. As a result, I proposed the most outrageous thing my intern therapist brain could conjure.

"What if we go over to the window and you tell me which building is the size of your terror?"

She giggled. "Ok, why not?"

We went over to the window together but no building outside the therapy room was big enough, she said, not even all of them put together. Yet the act of getting up and visually comparing physical buildings appeared to give my young client a thought.

"You know, it's more like my terror is so big that all the space outside this office isn't big enough for it." She waved her hand in front of the window. Then she looked at me. "It's like the terror is invading even this room. Like there's barely enough room in here for us."

She was smiling and excited, as if she'd found a treasure.

"Really?" I said. "So if the terror is invading this room too, where do you and I need to be?"

"Well, we'd be squished up against the wall."

"Let's try it, and see how that feels."

With her direction, we shoved ourselves into a corner together, shoulder to shoulder.

"Yes, this feels right," she said with a satisfied smile on her face. My client had just demonstrated the experience of intrusion (Herman, 1997), in which a person's present moment experience is eclipsed by the feelings and flashbacks of the trauma. As long as her feelings were unquantifiable, she felt like they had power over her. But by metaphorically quantifying them, she tasted a moment of mastery*, in which she gained some power over her traumatic experience. Though she had told me the story of her rape a few sessions before, simply telling the story had not brought much relief. Her trauma had less power over her when she allowed herself to feel the feelings of trauma in her body in the present moment experience. By standing in the corner of the room with me as if crowded by the trauma, she was enacting the invading quality of these feelings. After this enactment, we sat down and she told me what the experience was like. She looked and reported feeling lighter, especially in her chest. This was not a small thing: Before this moment she could not locate feelings in her body, now she could. She was reclaiming her own experience. As she consciously integrated the traumatic experience, and the toll it had exacted on her body and mind, she was also becoming more aware of her bodily sensations. Though her terror remained throughout our sessions together, she said it did not invade the room as it did on that first day.*

The vignette above demonstrates how vital incorporating the body is to trauma-focused therapy. Though yoga therapy was not used in this session, the client and I physically enacted her feelings. Many trauma experts agree that trauma therapy must include the body to be effective (Herman, 1997; Levine, 1997; van der Kolk, 2003). For this reason, yoga therapy may be an ideal adjunctive modality in trauma-focused therapy (Emerson & Hopper, 2011; Spinazzola et al., 2011; Interlandi, 2014).

To understand the ways that yoga therapy fits hand-in-glove with current trauma treatment, this chapter explores current definitions of trauma, childhood trauma and developmental trauma, yoga's role in the treatment and healing of trauma, a case study, a chapter summary of yoga therapy for trauma symptoms, and practices for trauma.

Defining trauma

According to the American Psychiatric Association (2014) *posttraumatic stress disorder* (PTSD) or *psychological trauma* occurs when an individual directly experiences or witnesses an event that one's body interprets as life threatening with no recourse available. Psychological trauma is experienced physically as well as emotionally, even when no harm is done to the body (Rothschild, 2000). This is because the body remains frozen in the physiological response of fear long after the cause of the fear is gone (Herman, 1997; Levine, 1997). Thus my client's experience of terror invading the therapy room was a traumatic response to being raped. Her body was stuck in the all-encompassing terror she had felt while it was happening.

Beyond the literal threat of death or bodily harm, being deeply humiliated or shamed may also cause trauma. In a 2014 interview (Appendix), Erica Viggiano said, "Any experience that creates a sense of annihilation or severe threat to the integrity of the self can cause trauma" (p. 122). As a licensed clinical social worker and registered yoga teacher, Viggiano has been using yoga for many years as a psychotherapy intervention with adults and adjudicated youth. Viggiano says that many trauma survivors have experienced both life-threatening trauma and a range of traumatic experiences and conditions that have compromised their sense of self, safety and competency in their own bodies, and therefore in the world they live in.

I too have witnessed how shame or bullying can cause extreme stress in children and adolescents in particular. For example, Jessica, whose story was featured in Chapter 3 on mood regulation issues, endured bullying and aggression from older girls on her high school basketball team when she was a freshman. Though she decided to take on their tough demeanor and fight back, she began suffering from panic attacks and severe stomach migraines that sent her to the emergency department. She told me she felt as if she had to fight back to survive. Her panic attacks appeared to be a symptom of how threatened she felt at school.

The neurobiology of traumatic memories

To understand trauma, it is important to understand how traumatic memories are stored in the brain and throughout the body. There are two kinds of memory—explicit and implicit (Cherry, 2014). An explicit memory is consciously and intentionally remembered information, such as recalling one's phone number. An implicit memory is unconscious and unintentional, and includes remembering tasks like swinging a baseball bat or riding a bike. Research shows that trauma seems to interfere with explicit memory while leaving implicit memories intact (van der Kolk, 1994; Rothschild, 2000). This means that the body sensations and visual images from trauma stay locked in the body, while the conscious recall of what happened is lost or distorted. This is often a disorienting and disturbing experience for individuals. The distortions or loss of explicit memory may have something to do with the neurobiology of trauma. Our current understanding of the neurobiology of trauma is that the neocortex of the brain's frontal lobe becomes disengaged during a traumatic event (van der Kolk, 1994). Simultaneously, the brainstem or limbic system becomes activated (Figure 4.1). This is an adaptive process in which the brain bypasses the thinking mind (e.g. the neocortex) in favor of the faster processing of the limbic system that decides whether the individual needs to fight, flee or freeze.

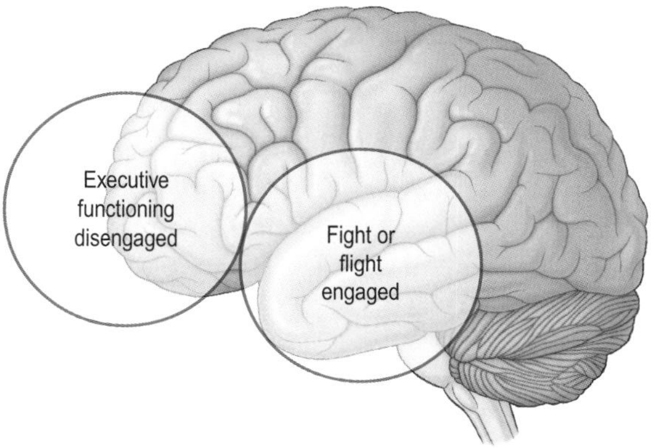

Figure 4.1
The neurobiology of trauma: The thinking mind (the prefrontal cortex) disengages, and the limbic system is activated to prepare the body for the fight, flight or freeze response

As a result, trauma treatment needs to include somatic interventions to help release the individual from the grips of traumatic memories (Levine, 1997; Rothschild, 2000; van der Kolk, 2009). My client from the vignette demonstrated that physically moving the body is essential to working through traumatic memories, which are also stored physically. Yoga therapy may be a particularly effective intervention, because its calming practices may help a traumatized individual regulate the disturbing process of remembering a traumatic event. These practices also give the individual the opportunity to learn to regulate their emotional and physical experiences independently, giving rise to a greater degree of self-mastery and personal effectiveness (Viggiano, 2014, personal communication).

Behavioral sequelae

Levine (1997) has referred to PTSD as shock trauma, which he says is "an external force rupturing the protective container . . . of our experience" (p. 197). The "protective container" that Levine refers to is one's sense of psychological and bodily safety in the world. PTSD shatters this sense of safety (Herman, 1997; Levine, 1997; van der Kolk, 2003). The individual suffering from PTSD will behave in ways to avoid, minimize or in some other way cope with her psycho-physiological triggers, sometimes consciously and sometimes unconsciously. The behaviors that result from PTSD are so central to the diagnosis that the American Psychiatric Association (2013) amended its definition in the DSM-5 to focus attention on four sets of behavioral symptoms: re-experiencing, avoidance, negative cognitions and mood, and arousal.

Because the neurobiology of trauma is complex, and the behavioral sequelae vary from individual to individual, both topics are covered more fully in the later sections of this chapter. Behavioral sequelae are covered in Intrusion versus constriction, while the neurobiology of trauma is covered more fully in Fight, flight, freeze.

Childhood trauma

The above depiction of trauma is based on our current understanding of adult PTSD. Not surprisingly, psychological trauma experienced in childhood is different to trauma experienced as an adult (Briere, 1992; Herman, 1997 ; Rothschild, 2000; Perry, 2009). This is because trauma that happens in childhood occurs when an individual is still developing on all levels—physically, psychologically, emotionally and mentally (Briere, 1992). The earlier a trauma occurs in a child's life, the greater the chance of negative long-term effects, such as psychopathology (Herman, 1997).

The National Child Traumatic Stress Network (NCTSN) lists 13 types of childhood traumas: community, complex, domestic violence, early childhood, medical, natural disasters, neglect, physical abuse, refugee and war zone trauma, school violence, sexual abuse, terrorism, and traumatic grief (NCTSN, 2013). This list reflects a growing awareness in the field that childhood trauma can be complex, especially since it occurs during a child's development and may be chronic. One of the most critical aspects of development over the course of childhood is developing a sense of self, and trauma interrupts this developing self in ways we have yet to understand.

Developmental trauma

In 2009 Bessel van der Kolk and colleagues proposed a new diagnosis of developmental trauma disorder be added to the DSM-V, which was subsequently published in 2013. Developmental trauma disorder is not included in the DSM-5. However, van der Kolk and colleagues made a salient point in their proposal paper, "Whether or not they exhibit symptoms of PTSD, children who have developed in the context of ongoing danger, maltreatment, and inadequate caregiving systems are ill-served by the current diagnostic system . . ." (p. 2).

Children who are exposed to maltreatment, family violence, and other chronic forms of trauma often meet criteria for a laundry list of DSM-5 diagnoses including depression, anxiety, ADHD, ODD, conduct disorders, eating disorders, sleep disorders, attachment issues, and physical illness and complications (Briere, 1992; Herman, 1997; Cook et al., 2005). Given the intersection of developmental trauma with such an array of mental health diagnoses, it is helpful to understand how trauma affects one's behavior and disrupts one's ability to self-regulate emotional states.

Intrusion versus constriction

In her landmark book *Trauma and Recovery* (1997), Judith Herman introduced the concept of the dialectic of trauma, in which an individual vacillates between symptoms of intrusion and constriction. She says that the trauma victim finds herself "caught between the extremes of amnesia or of reliving the trauma" (p. 47). Intrusive symptoms include flashbacks (or re-experiencing), insomnia, panic attacks, unnecessary risk taking, and hyperarousal (Herman, 1997; Levine, 1997). A classic example of flashback/re-experiencing is of a war veteran who hears a car backfire, and instinctively drops to the pavement. He is not responding with his conscious awareness. Instead, his nervous system registers the sound of the backfiring car as gunfire. Hyper-arousal occurs when an individual has a hyper vigilant startle response, or seems constantly to be on edge.

On the other hand, constrictive symptoms include a trance-like, spacey or flat affect, as well as avoidance of certain situations or people (Herman, 1997; Levine, 1997; Rothschild, 2000). Substance abuse is a common way for trauma sufferers to dull unwanted sensations, feelings and flashbacks. Another common symptom of constriction is dissociation, a numbed state in which the individual may appear and actually report a sense of detached calm (Herman, 1997). Dissociation causes changes in perception, such as time slowing, feeling "checked out" from the present moment, or even amnesia.

Vacillating from constriction to intrusion does not help the individual heal from or integrate the traumatic event into his life. Instead, he rides the roller coaster of these two extremes. To understand the internal landscape of those suffering from PTSD, researchers and clinicians have turned to neuroscience to understand its effects on the brain and nervous system.

Fight, flight, freeze

Imagine a very powerful sports car. The nervous system at rest is like that sports car sitting idle—it has a lot of potential, but it uses minimal energy. When an individual is in the midst of an intrusive state of PTSD, it is as if she is gunning the engine suddenly. In contrast, when she dissociates (i.e. in the midst of a constrictive state), she is both gunning the engine while slamming on the brakes. In other words, dissociation expends a lot of energy. The symptoms of PTSD tax the nervous system tremendously. Babette Rothschild explains this process in *The Body Remembers* (2000):

"People with PTSD live with a chronic state of . . . hyper arousal . . . in their bodies, leading to physical symptoms that are the basis of anxiety, panic, weakness, exhaustion, muscle stiffness, concentration problems, and sleep disturbance" (p. 47).

During extreme stress or threat, the nervous system responds instinctively—and without an individual's conscious will—by activating the *autonomic nervous system*, or the ANS (Rothschild, 2000). During this state of hyper-arousal, the brain releases hormones that prepare the body for action. If the ANS deems fight or flight possible, it will activate the sympathetic nervous system resulting in increased heart rate, dilated pupils, pale skin (as the blood migrates toward the internal organs), and quickened motor response, along with other mobilizing actions. If there is no possibility of escape, the ANS will trigger not only the sympathetic nervous system but the parasympathetic nervous system as well, causing immobility in the limbs. (This is the gunning the engine while slamming on the brakes.) It is also the freeze response seen in a prey animal that "plays dead" when no escape is possible from its predator (Herman, 1997; Levine, 1997; Rothschild, 2000; van der Kolk, 2009).

A gazelle that has nearly been gored by a lion will shake violently, releasing lactic acid build-up in its muscles that cause the freeze response (Levine, 1997). The lactic acid build-up mimics rigor mortis, which tricks the predator into thinking the gazelle is dead. But the process of recovery is not so simple for humans. An individual suffering from PTSD is literally "stuck" in the freeze response (Levine, 1997), due to the neural circuitry of trauma. "Neuroimaging studies of human beings in highly emotional states reveal that intense emotions, such as anger, fear or sadness, cause increased activity in the brain regions related to fear and self-preservation and reduced activity in the brain regions related to feeling fully present" (van der Kolk, 2009, p. 12). Thus, the individual does not shake off the physical chemicals associated with extreme stress. In addition, he also has a harder time emotionally and cognitively attending to life after the stress is over.

Yoga and trauma

Trauma is stored in the body. Thus, yoga fits well with current evidenced based models of trauma treatment. "If you practice yoga and can develop a body that is strong and feels comfortable, this can contribute substantially to help you come into the here and now rather than staying stuck in the past" (van der Kolk, 2009, p. 12).

Bessel van der Kolk (2009) suggests that the intensity of some yoga postures may be the key to yoga's effectiveness in the treatment of trauma. Intense postures illicit strong physical responses such as faster heart rate and breathing, sweating, and muscular stretching or contraction. Such action-oriented practice may help an individual release chronically tense muscles associated with the trauma, and allow the individual to engage in an effective physical response. Viggiano (2014) says she draws upon action-oriented practices like diaphragmatic breathing, yoga or martial arts with her clients to give them a sense of physical effectiveness and self-directedness.

Intense physical practice can also lead to a growing sense of mastery and control of overwhelming bodily experiences. In her book *Fierce Medicine* (2011) yoga master Ana Forrest recalls her own experience of using intense physical practice to heal from trauma. Despite her fear of heights, she jumped off a high ledge into a river multiple times:

" . . . I'd clamber all the way up and just jump right away so the fear wouldn't have time to build, the paralysis wouldn't deepen, and all the subterranean scary stories in my head couldn't bubble up. I didn't wait to feed the fear. I just took a deep breath, exhaled, and jumped. The fear was there, but it wasn't unmanageable. I'd believed that in order to do what I was afraid of, I had to get rid of the fear first, but that turned out to be only an idea, not the truth" (p. 10).

Trauma-sensitive yoga

Safe and effective trauma-sensitive yoga occurs when the intentions for the session are communicated effectively through the instructions. The yoga program at the Trauma Center at Justice Resource Institute (JRI) in Boston, MA, recommends some key themes for trauma-sensitive yoga: experiencing the present moment, making choices, taking effective action, and creating rhythms. Experiencing the present moment is accomplished through attention to somatic sensations while practicing deep breathing and asana. The yoga therapist encourages the student(s) to make choices by giving options. For instance, the practice sequence included in *Overcoming Trauma through Yoga* (Emerson & Hopper, 2011) offers different options of body position for most poses.

The reason choice is so important in trauma-sensitive yoga therapy is that individuals are robbed of the ability to make choices for their bodies or themselves while in the midst of a traumatic event. By allowing an individual as many choices as possible in yoga therapy, the individual physically enacts her ability to make choices and take back her power.

Trauma-sensitive yoga instruction is languaged quite differently than in an average yoga class. Rather than pushing students to challenge themselves more, the yoga therapist uses "invitational language emphasizing gentle exploration of bodily movements and associated physical sensations" (Spinazzola et al., 2011, p. 436). Instructions such as "If you would like..." or "you may experience..." encourage a student to gently become aware of his internal body sensations. Once a student can tolerate his present moment sensation and is given choices, he can take effective action. For instance, he can choose a different arm position in a pose if he feels discomfort or pain. The JRI has also found that the repetitive movements of some yoga poses "appear to restore and entrain the rhythmicity of biological functions that are often disrupted during periods of stress" (Salmon et al., 2009, p. 62).

Rothschild's Braking and Accelerating

Returning to the car metaphor used earlier, trauma treatment is like learning to drive a powerful sports car (Rothschild, 2000). If one wants a smooth ride, one must first learn to put on the brakes before accelerating. "It is inadvisable for a therapist to accelerate trauma processes in clients or for a client to accelerate toward his own trauma, until each first knows how to hit the brakes" (p. 79). Rothschild's car metaphor parallels Herman's dialectic of trauma; by learning to hit the brakes in the therapeutic process, the client begins to take control of the roller coaster of intrusive and constrictive symptoms.

In yoga therapy, "hitting the brakes" may mean one of several things: doing an easier version of a triggering pose, coming out of the triggering pose and doing a safe pose, stopping asana practice to focus on breathing, or taking a break from any kind of somatic practice. In this scenario, a triggering pose is any pose that a client says triggers his thoughts, feelings, sensations or flashbacks related to the trauma. A safe pose is any pose (or poses) that an individual has already deemed comforting and relaxing.

Thus, the first step in yoga therapy is for the client to determine his safe poses. This first crucial step is where a client learns to replace constrictive behaviors and symptoms with conscious, intentional behaviors. The next step occurs as he becomes more comfortable in the yoga practice: He is able to hold poses that once were triggering. By spending a limited, prescribed amount of time in a challenging yoga posture, the individual discovers that "he can tolerate intense sensation . . . In essence, his body becomes safe again" (van der Kolk, 2009). In this way, yoga (or any somatic technique) can facilitate the overall therapeutic process and even make it less volatile (Rothschild, 2000).

Accelerating occurs when a client either inadvertently or intentionally experiences triggering thoughts, emotions or sensations. When this happens accidentally, the yoga therapist coaches the client to use his safe poses or other calming practices. When used intentionally, this therapeutic technique is a form of exposure therapy. Exposure therapy requires special training, and therefore is not covered in this chapter.

The NCTSN says that some of the essential components of trauma treatment are safety, self-regulation, and traumatic experience integration (Cook et al., 2005). Yoga therapy for trauma empowers an individual to get in touch with thoughts, emotions and feelings from which he once distanced himself for fear of triggering traumatic memories. Viggiano (2014) says that yoga can provide a safe environment in which the individual can begin to "befriend" his experience with present moment awareness. Practices that cultivate mindful awareness help the individual discover that each moment comes to an end in the transition to the next moment. For example, when an individual practices deep breathing he discovers that the inhale ends as the exhalation begins. As he becomes reacquainted (or perhaps acquainted for the first time) with his internal body sensations, he learns he has some control. It is this very process that can empower a traumatized individual to integrate the traumatic experiences (experienced as present moment body sensations) into his current life narrative.

"What is beautiful about yoga is that it teaches us . . . that things come to an end" (van der Kolk, 2009, p. 13).

Case study: The disappearing act

A 15-year-old girl was admitted to the eating disorder unit for very low weight and signs of eating disorder behavior. Although she was emaciated like her peers, she did not shake and fidget trying to burn calories like they did. Instead, she sat quite still at the back of her yoga mat in her first yoga group with her arms wrapped around her legs. Her demeanor seemed flat yet defiant, versus the usually bright and pleasing affect of many eating disorder patients. She privately shared with another staff member that she had been raped a year ago.

I received an individual referral for yoga therapy with her. To create an atmosphere of safety in our first individual session, I followed her lead as much as possible. I asked her to find the most comfortable position to sit in as we talked about her goals for yoga therapy and decided what poses to do together. She complained that she did not know how she felt most of the time, until she felt suicidal or wanted to self-harm. She did know she hated herself

Case studies *(Continued)*

most of the time, and felt like she was "fat." As she told me these things she sat with her arms around her knees, much like she had in the group yoga sessions. I reflected this to her gently, and she shared that this contracted sitting position and *balasana* made her feel safe. I invited her to do *balasana* with me. Once we were in the pose, I asked her how she felt.

"It feels good, comforting," she replied.

"Well, congratulations, because you just identified how you feel—comfortable."

She laughed a little at this.

She decided her goal for yoga therapy was to become aware of what she was feeling in the present moment, and then learn how to respond to it. I used the practice sequence from *Overcoming Trauma through Yoga: Reclaiming Your Body* (Emerson & Hopper, 2011). She chose *balasana* as her safe pose any time she felt triggered or uncomfortable in another pose. Sweeping her arms up overhead seemed to be one of the more triggering moves for her. Over time she became more proficient at labeling her experience, using the different poses to notice different sensations. I encouraged her to try different variations of poses to figure out what felt best. In this way, she learned how to self-regulate her somatic experience.

After our sessions, she reported feeling more relaxed and at home in her body. I observed that she looked more alive and animated, and she agreed. The dullness faded from her eyes, which sparkled more, and she could label body sensations more easily (though emotions were still difficult for her). I did not tell her that the sequence we practiced was specifically designed for trauma suffers. In fact, we didn't talk about her rape until she brought it up in our fifth session together. It is best practice to wait to talk about a patient's trauma until after several sessions. Once she has identified and can readily use her safe pose(s), she will be able to self-regulate more readily. Before talking about the narrative at all, it is best to explain Rothchild's "hitting the brakes" philosophy and how it applies to yoga practice.

In summary

Yoga therapy may be an excellent adjunct therapy in comprehensive trauma treatment. Because trauma is stored physically in somatic memory, the body is essential in treating trauma. Practicing trauma-sensitive yoga may help the individual suffering from trauma release traumatic memories stored in the body in a safe and self-regulating fashion.

Children who experience chronic trauma over the course of their development may suffer from developmental trauma, a term being used by some trauma experts to describe the lasting effects of trauma disguised as other symptoms. While behavioral symptoms of anxiety and depression (as well as a host of other sequelae) must be addressed, treatment is incomplete if the source of these behavioral symptoms is trauma and it remains unrecognized and untreated. Yoga therapy may be especially helpful for this population who have not learned basic skills of self-regulation.

Yoga also fits well with current models of trauma treatment, which focus on coping skills and self-regulation through somatic experiencing. Armed with Rothschild's "hitting the brakes" approach and tools from the JRI yoga program, a yoga therapist is well-equipped to empower patients with trauma to reconnect and feel safe in their bodies.

Practice considerations

As mentioned earlier, individuals with trauma benefit when they are given choices. Thus, the first principle when designing a yoga sequence or intervention for trauma is to offer as much choice as possible. My own approach to giving a child choice is to help him determine his "safe pose" or other safe yoga techniques that he can come back to when he needs to self-regulate. Doing this explicitly is more important for school-aged or younger children, who are concrete thinkers. Adolescents may not need this much structure, but still need to be given plenty of choice.

Because choice is so important in trauma-sensitive yoga, the practices below are suggestions, and not prescriptions. Attuning with a child or adolescent's specific needs and collaborating with him or her will help a yoga therapist not only develop an effective, individualized yoga practice but also establish a supportive relationship with the child.

Lastly, because trauma survivors often have individual needs, these practices are written with an individual yoga session in mind, versus a group experience.

Training resources

Whether working in a large institution or in private practice, a yoga therapist should obtain as much trauma-sensitive training as possible before working with client who suffer with trauma. In addition to reading Emerson and Hopper's book on trauma-sensitive yoga treatment, *Overcoming Trauma through Yoga* (2011), one can find educational resources online. The NCTSN website offers a plethora of resources regarding complex trauma education and treatment: www.nctsn.org. Attending conferences and workshops can also bolster yoga therapists' skills. In 2014, the National Kid Yoga Conference featured two presentations on yoga for children and adolescents with trauma: Yoga-Based Psychotherapy for Children Who Have Experienced Trauma and Neglect, presented by the Kennedy Krieger Institute, and Children, Trauma, and Exposure to Violence: The Use of Yoga and Mindfulness as Healing Modalities, presented by NYU Langone Medical Center and others.

Models of trauma treatment

Recall Herman's dialectic of trauma, in which the PTSD symptoms of intrusion and constriction carry the victim on a psychological and physical roller coaster ride. The ultimate goal of trauma-focused treatment is to empower the individual to unwind herself from the ups and downs of this cycle to once again (or perhaps for the first time) feel connected and safe in her body (Spinazzola et al., 2011). Healing from trauma of any kind is a slow, stepwise and often complicated process (Cook et al., 2005). Thus, it is helpful to keep this essential goal in mind.

In trauma treatment, developing coping skills occurs before addressing traumatic memories. Marylene Cloitre has developed the Skills Training in Affective and Interpersonal Regulation (STAIR) model of complex trauma treatment, in which coping skills are taught before addressing the trauma narrative (Emerson & Hopper, 2011).

School-aged children

School-aged and younger children need structure as well as choice when starting yoga practice. One way the yoga therapist can create structure is to set up the room before the child's arrival (e.g. clear a space if the room is used for other purposes, set out mats, lower the lights, and any other environmental modifications that will facilitate a calm atmosphere). Another way to create structure is to use a set of yoga flashcards from which the child can choose poses for practice. Especially in the first few sessions,

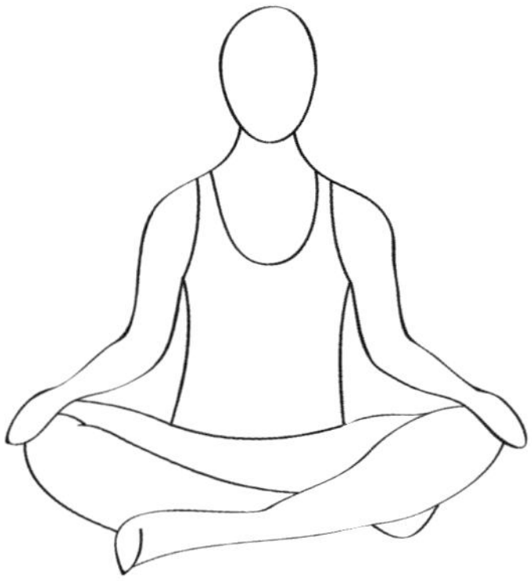

Figure 4.2
Sukhasana (Simple Sitting Pose) with arm raises (3–5 times)

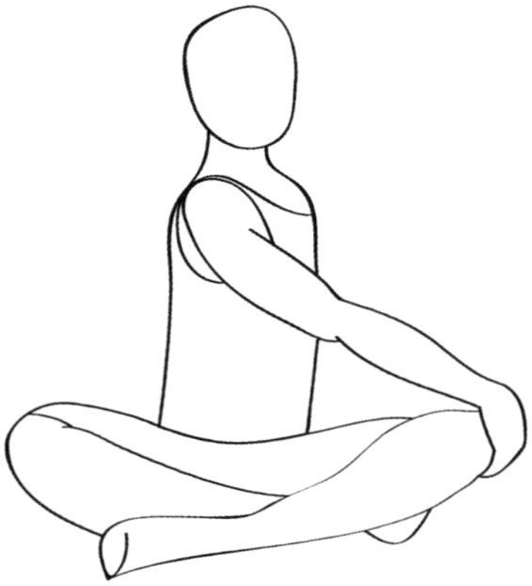

Figure 4.3
Sukhasana Twist (Seated Twist)—repeat on both sides

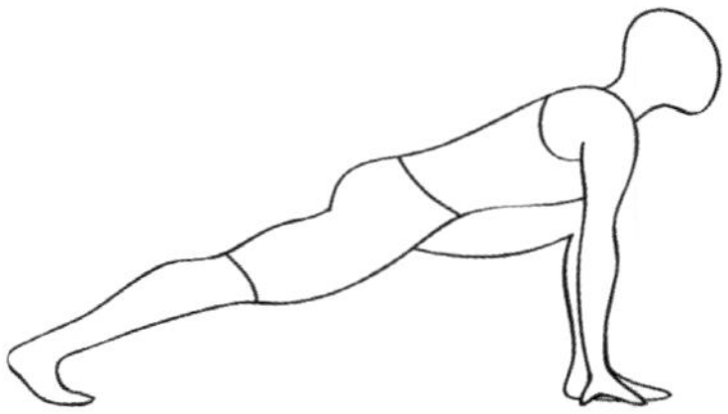

Figure 4.4
Lunge—repeat on both sides

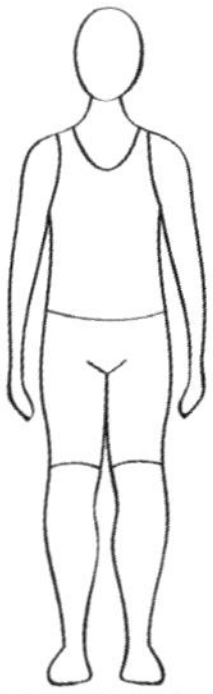

Figure 4.5
Tadasana (Mountain Pose)

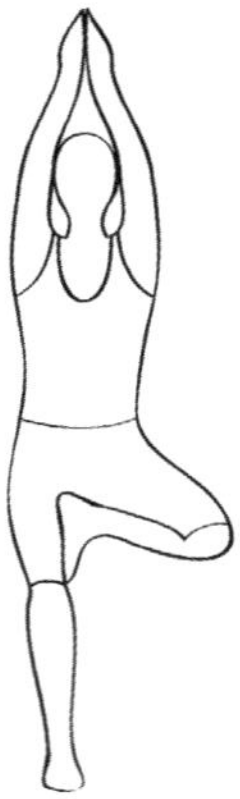

Figure 4.6
Vrksasana (Tree Pose)—repeat on both sides

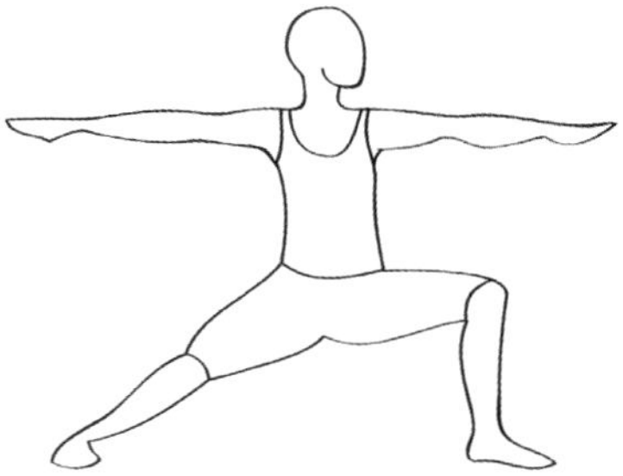

Figure 4.7
Virabhadrasana II (Warrior II)—repeat on both sides

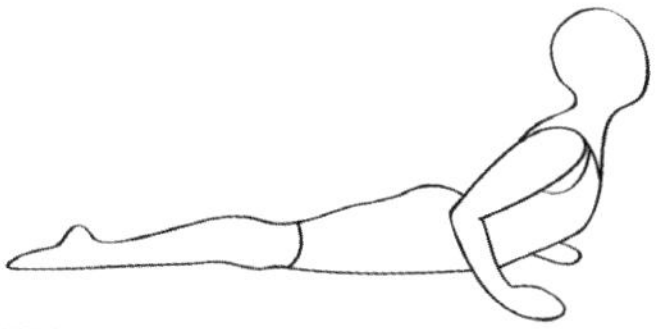

Figure 4.8
Bhujangasana (Cobra Pose)

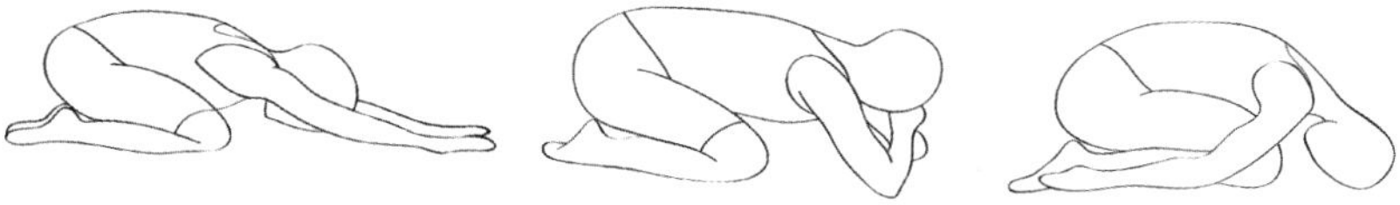

Figure 4.9A, B & C
Pick a variation of Balasana (Child's Pose)

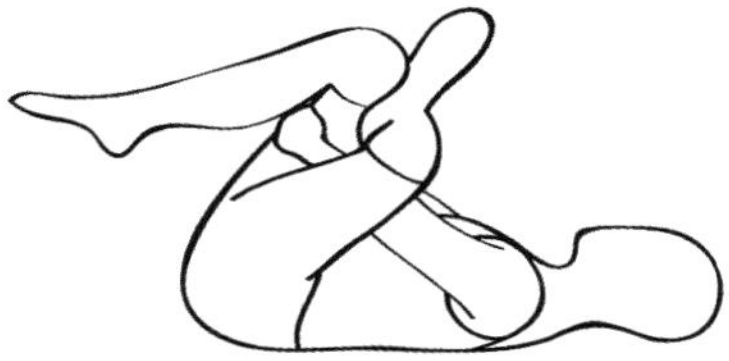

Figure 4.10
Sucirandhra (Eye of the Needle Pose)—repeat on both sides Sa Ta Na Ma mantra or Counting Breaths

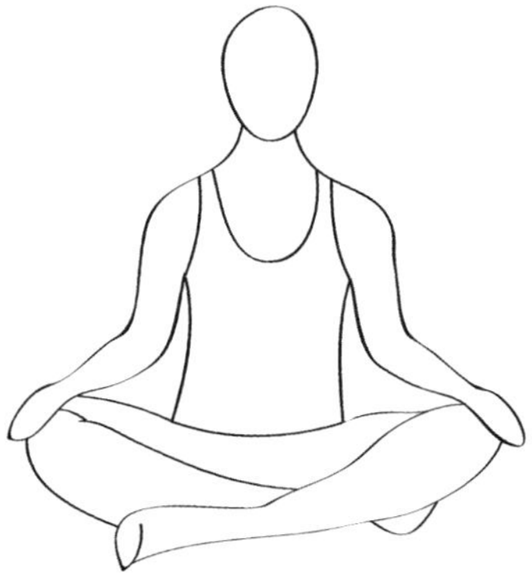

Figure 4.11
Sukhasana (Simple Sitting Pose) with arm raises (3–5 times)

a shorter length session is best as the child becomes familiar with yoga practice. I find 30–45 minutes is ideal for many school-aged children. During this time, we may do anywhere from five to ten yoga poses and techniques. Refer to Chapter 9 for detailed instructions, modifications and contraindications of the poses.

Ring a bell to indicate the beginning of the yoga therapy session.

Adolescents

This sequence is based on the case study in this chapter. In contrast to the child's practice, this one involves much less movement. The focus of our practices was more on choice-making and observing body sensations than big movements.

Ring a bell to indicate the beginning of the yoga therapy session.

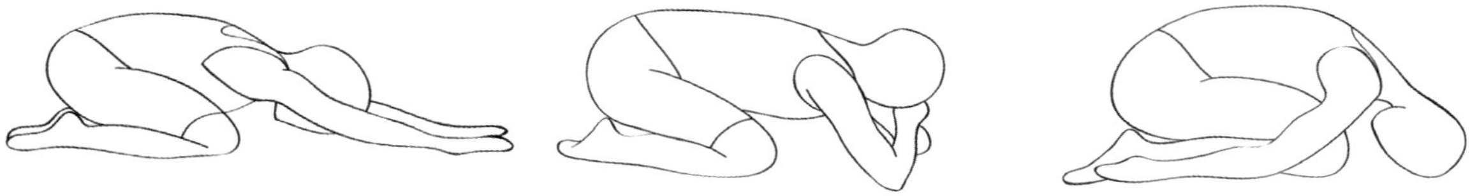

Figure 4.12 A, B & C
Pick a variation of Balasana (Child's Pose)

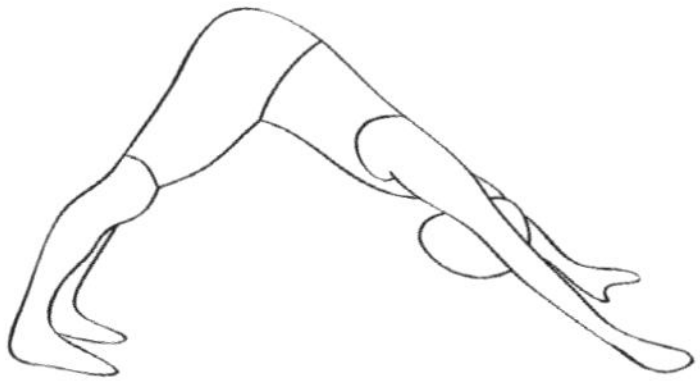

Figure 4.13
Adho Mukha Svanasana (Downward-facing Dog Pose)

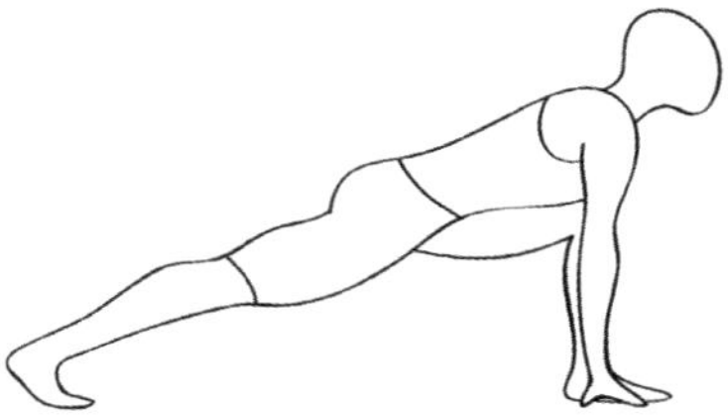

Figure 4.14
Lunge—repeat on both sides

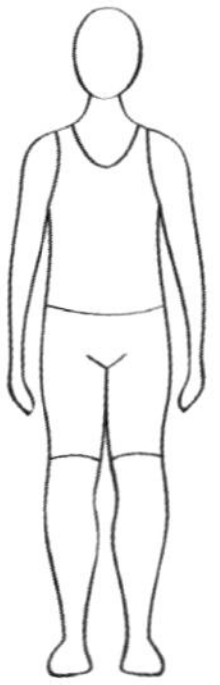

Figure 4.15
Tadasana (Mountain Pose)

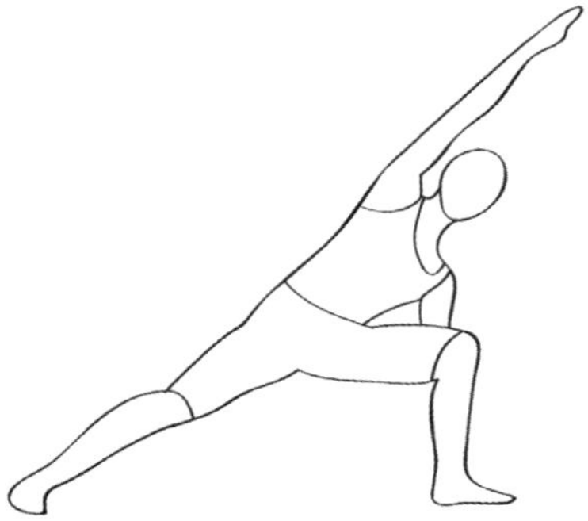

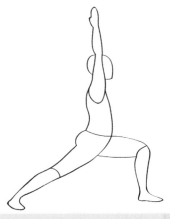

Figure 4.16
Utthita Parsvakonasana (Side Angle Stretch)

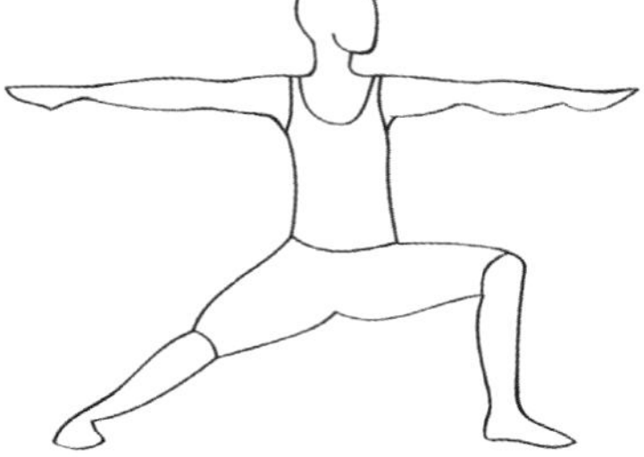

Figure 4.17
Virabhadrasana II (Warrior II)—repeat on both sides

Figure 4.18
Virabhadrasana I (Warrior I)—repeat on both sides

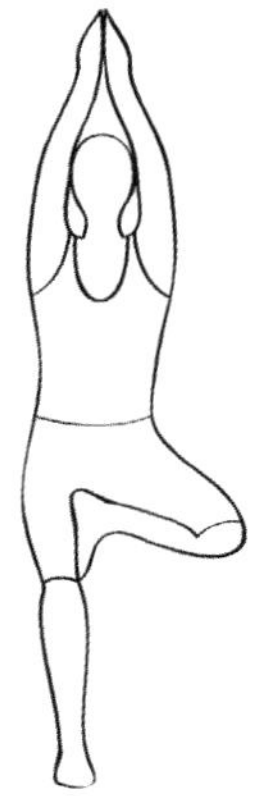

Figure 4.19
Vrksasana (Tree Pose)—repeat on both sides

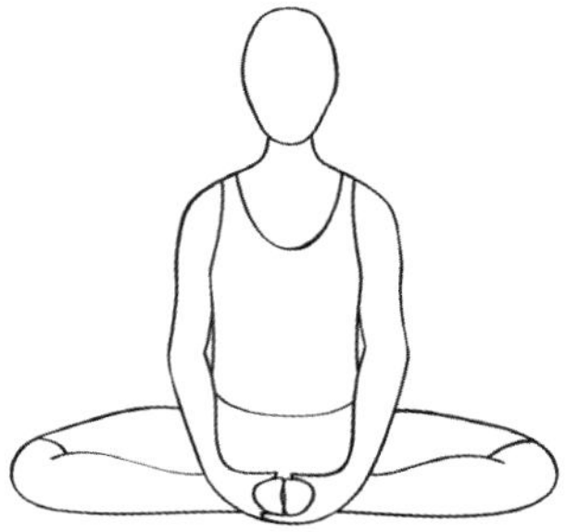

Figure 4.20
Baddha Konasana (Cobbler's Pose)

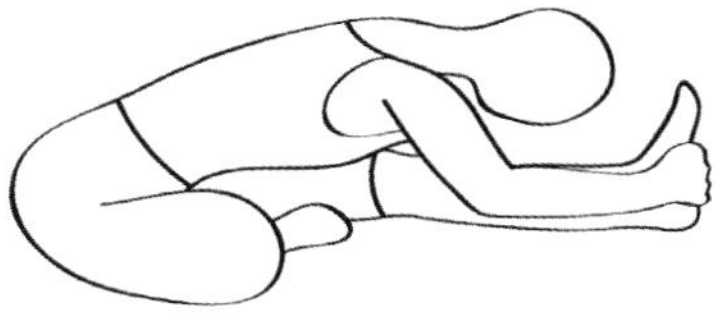

Figure 4.21
Janu Sirsasana (Runner's Stretch Pose)—repeat on both sides

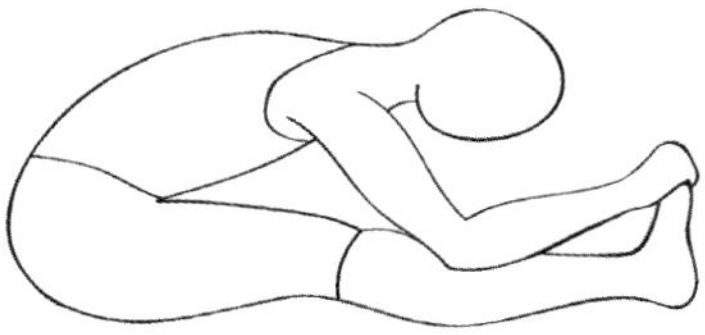

Figure 4.22
Paschimottanasana (Seated Forward Fold)

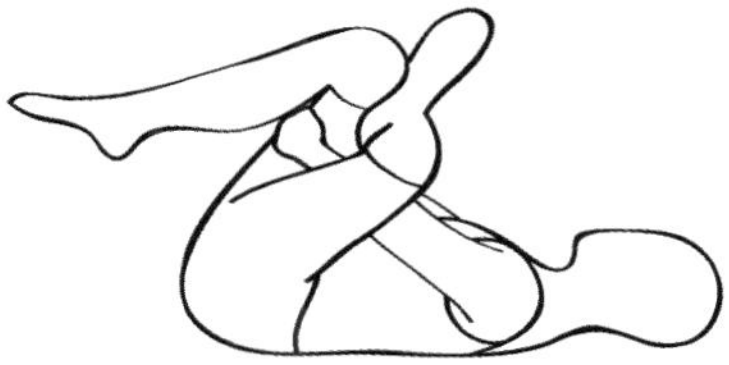

Figure 4.23
Sucirandhra (Eye of the Needle Pose)—repeat on both sides

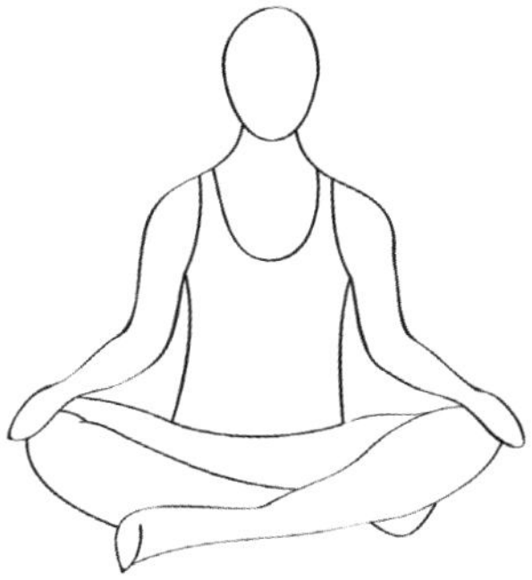

Figure 4.24
Sitting in Sukhasana, practice Sa Ta Na Ma mantra or Counting Breaths

Sa Ta Na Ma Mantra

This is best for adolescents but some school-aged children may also enjoy it.

- Sit up tall, but relaxed. Notice the breath coming in and going out.
- Bring thumbs and index fingers together and say "Sa"
- Bring thumbs and middle fingers together and say "Ta"
- Bring thumbs and ring fingers together and say "Na"
- Bring thumbs and pinkie fingers together and say "Ma"
- Repeat 5–10 times

Try slowing the last few repetitions down even further, and notice what happens to the speed of your thoughts and your state of mind.

Counting Breath (for school-aged children and adolescents)

- Notice the breath coming in and going out
- Inhale, notice the expansive, opening, lengthening qualities of the inhale
- Exhale, notice the dropping, rooting, grounding qualities of the exhale
- Notice that the breath naturally slows down as you bring awareness to it
- Count how long your next inhalation is
- Exhale, to the same count
- Every time the mind wanders, just bring it back to the simple count of the breath
- School-aged children can do this practice for up to a minute; adolescents can do it for up to 5 minutes

Eating Disorders and Body Image Issues

5

Brownies as scary as skydiving: A few years ago, a father of a girl with an eating disorder shared an epiphany about his daughter's condition with other struggling parents. In the eating disorder multi-family group I co-facilitate, this father told the other parents in the group that he saw the look of terror on his daughter's face when he placed a brownie in front of her as part of her meal plan. He said as he watched her face, he realized that the fearful reaction she had to the brownie reminded him of his own fear of heights. In that moment, he said, he stopped trying to figure out why the brownie terrified her, and instead realized he'd be just as terrified as her if someone asked him to jump out of a plane. He'd noticed that sometimes in their hotel room his daughter would actually put her hands over her ears as if there was too much noise in her head. In the same way, he said that if he were about to jump from a plane, there'd probably be a lot of noise from the engines. So the person instructing him to jump would have to use a firm but warm tone of voice to engender trust and confidence in him.

This father modeled the kind of non-judgmental compassion and empathy that is needed when trying to understand a child's eating disorder. After that group, many parents said the father's skillful analogy helped them reassess their view of their own child's eating disorder. They could stop asking the question "why" and instead have compassion for their child's fears, no matter how inexplicable the fears seemed to them.

Eating disorders (ED) and ED behaviors are complex. They are often comorbid with other symptoms and diagnoses, such as OCD, anxiety, depression, and substance abuse (Steiner et al., 2003; Lock & le Grange, 2005; Klein & Cook-Cottone, 2013).

The mere presence of an eating disorder can be life threatening in a way that no other mental health diagnosis is (National Association of Anorexia Nervosa and Associated Disorders, 2014). Additionally, EDs present differently in children and adolescents than in adults. Further, they present differently in boys versus girls. Given the complexity of pediatric eating disorders it is important to bring the same level of compassion and empathy to a child struggling with an eating disorder as the father in the vignette showed his daughter. I work with patients, families and staff on the Eating Disorders Unit (EDU) at Children's Hospital Colorado, which places a strong emphasis on the family component.

Yoga therapy is a great adjunctive therapy in eating disorder treatment, because it helps the child, parents, and treating clinicians focus on compassion and empathy rather than asking "why." To understand the multi-faceted nature of a pediatric eating disorder and how yoga therapy aids in its overall treatment, we will consider

1) what an eating disorder is
2) who is prone to EDs and ED behavior, and
3) the ways in which yoga therapy can minimize ED risk factors and bolster ED protective factors.

Current literature on yoga and eating disorders will be discussed throughout this section. The fourth section in this chapter will feature two case studies to illustrate the principles presented. And finally, the fifth section contains a few practice sessions to demonstrate how to put the principles into practice.

What is an eating disorder?

The National Eating Disorder Association (2015) defines eating disorders as "serious emotional and physical problems that can have life-threatening consequences." The current wisdom is that an eating disorder is an expression of an individual's desire to gain control, when she feels like she has none (Steiner et al., 2003; Lock & le Grange, 2005). Food becomes the object of control, whether it's over eating, under eating, binging and purging, or a combination of these. In this sense, an eating disorder is a crisis of mind and body, where the mind tries to control unwanted feelings by controlling food. Paradoxically, when eating patterns are severely altered over a period of time, the body adapts and alters brain chemistry, making the eating disordered behavior easier to maintain. (In the case of anorexia, this happens by the stomach shrinking, making the individual feel full sooner than is normal.) Thus, this mistaken strategy of controlling emotional states through physical means seems to work for the person with an eating disorder, for a while.

The DSM-5 identifies four main categories of eating disorders: Anorexia Nervosa (AN), Bulimia Nervosa (BN), Binge Eating Disorders and Eating Disorder Not Elsewhere Specified (ED NEC). Anorexia includes distorted body image and excessive dieting that results in significant weight loss and an obsessive fear of gaining weight. Bulimia is characterized by a binge/purge cycle. Though it's common for those with bulimia to purge via self-induced vomiting, purging can take the form of over exercising (either in addition to or instead of vomiting), laxative abuse, excessive exercising or fasting. Binge Eating Disorder is characterized by episodes of eating much more food in a short time period than is usual for most people, and includes feelings of being out of control. ED NEC replaces the DSM-IV term ED NOC (Eating Disorder Not Otherwise Specified), and is very similar in that it comprises a wide variety of disordered eating behaviors and thoughts, perhaps lacking in intensity, duration or physical markers necessary to warrant a full AN or BN diagnosis. In the past, the ED NOS was one of the more common diagnoses given to children and adolescents with eating disorders, because they often don't fit neatly into the diagnostic criteria of AN or BN (Steiner et al., 2003; Lock & le Grange, 2005).

Though obesity is a serious public health issue (especially in the United States), it is not an eating disorder in and of itself. The term *obesity* refers purely to physical characteristics of one's body mass index (BMI). Someone who is diagnosed as obese as a result of his BMI will only receive a diagnosis of an eating disorder if the reason(s) for the obesity falls within the diagnostic criteria of an eating disorder, such as ED NEC. Interestingly, some children and adolescents who had childhood obesity later develop an eating disorder—this is especially true for males who develop adolescent eating disorders. Obesity will be discussed in more detail in the two case studies in this chapter.

Treating a pediatric eating disorder

One of the thorniest issues in treating a pediatric eating disorder is that the diagnostic criteria for EDs are based on adult characteristics (Lock & le Grange, 2005). Because children and adolescents are still developing physically, the weight criteria and menstrual criteria are not appropriate for children or young adolescents, or males. In addition, younger patients tend to underreport the severity of their ED behaviors.

Another complex aspect of a pediatric eating disorder is the way in which it manifests as both an individual and a family issue. While the child has to be motivated enough to maintain her weight and good eating habits once in treatment, the family also plays a crucial role in the treatment and recovery of a child's or adolescent's eating disorder. In one treatment strategy called Family-Based Treatment (FBT), the family helps create structure through meal planning, and through other therapeutic skills they learn in treatment. Yet the individual child also needs to regain a sense of self-sufficiency and empowerment. As the father in the vignette described, a family's unconditional empathy can create a supportive, safe environment in which the child might regain a sense of trust and power again. (Whereas the vignette presents the father's viewpoint, case studies later in this chapter will feature children and adolescents' perspectives of an eating disorder.)

Who develops an eating disorder?

While issues of weight and diet are critical when considering ED and ED behavior, food intake is only part of the issue in an eating disorder. Current theory (Steiner et al., 2003; Lock & le Grange, 2005) holds that the core issue in an eating disorder may be an individual's sense of powerlessness and lack of control. Jarod, the 18-year-old male, mentioned in the Preface, demonstrated this powerlessness: He became anorexic during a time in his life when he felt many things were out of his control—his thwarted desire to play baseball as seriously as he wanted to, and his uncertainty about what he wanted to do after graduating from high school. He said yoga helped restore his self-confidence (personal communication, 2012).

What causes some bright young people like Jarod to fall prey to feelings of powerlessness and develop an eating disorder, while the vast majority of children and adolescents do not?

ED risk and protective factors: An introduction

Many ED prevention and treatment programs believe that *risk* and *protective factors* play a key role in whether a child develops symptoms of an eating disorder or not (Steiner et al., 2003; Lock & le Grange, 2005; Klein & Cook-Cottone, 2013). Risk factors such as low self-esteem and *body dissatisfaction* may increase the likelihood of an individual developing an eating disorder (Steiner et al., 2003; Klein & Cook-Cottone, 2013). Protective factors such as high self-esteem and a sense of self-competence may decrease that likelihood (Klein & Cook-Cottone, 2013). Steiner and colleagues (2003) postulated biological, psychological and social risk factors may play a role in the development of an eating disorder.

One particularly potent illustration of risk and protective factors came from a meta-analysis by Klein & Cook-Cottone (2013). These authors reviewed the extant literature on the effectiveness of yoga for eating disorders. The factors they postulate match well with my own experience of working with eating disorders. This review also happened to examine the other six studies found in an internet search conducted in March 2014, using three search engines (PubMed, PsychInfo, and GoogleScholar). It is worth noting that the Klein and Cook-Cottone review found 14 articles that met the following two criteria: 1) at least one yoga practice was used (such as pranayama, asana, relaxation or meditation), and 2) at least one ED outcome was measured. As mentioned in previous chapters, the RCT is the gold standard of research. Yet only three of these 14 studies were RCTs. The remainder were of less rigorous design (such as within-subjects and between-subjects designs).

Given the thoroughness and relevance of the Klein and Cook-Cottone review, I will use their list of factors to explore how yoga may be effective in the treatment of eating disorders. Their list of risk factors include:

1) body dissatisfaction
2) self-objectification
3) drive for thinness, and
4) body and emotional awareness.

The three protective factors for EDs noted by Klein and Cook-Cottone are:

1) self-competence
2) self-esteem, and
3) emotion regulation.

Yoga may reduce ED risk factors

Body dissatisfaction refers to negative body image. Klein and Cook-Cottone (2013) cite four studies (Daubenmeier, 2005; Dittman & Freedman, 2009; Delaney & Anthis, 2010; Zajac & Schier, 2011) that found that yoga practice seems to increase yoga practitioners' overall satisfaction with their bodies, whether or not the subjects were diagnosed with EDs. It appears that yoga classes that focus more on mind-body aspects of practice such as precise control of body, breathing, spiritual aspiration, or philosophical inquiry seemed especially effective in combatting body dissatisfaction.

Focusing on mind-body aspects of yoga seems to be an effective method for young people struggling with EDs. This risk factor can be addressed through an intervention I call "Body Sensations as Constellations," in which participants are asked to become aware of body sensations throughout the yoga session in a structured way. (This intervention is one of two featured practices at the end of this chapter.) At the beginning of yoga group, participants massage the soles of their feet with a tennis ball. After massaging their first foot, I stop them and ask them to notice the differences between feet. Generally, several participants notice that the foot they have just massaged feels looser, tingly, or simply has more sensation than the one they have not yet massaged. For the rest of the session, participants are invited to notice out loud where they feel sensations in different parts of their bodies. At the end of the group session a body scan can help integrate participants' experience.

A body scan inspired by Tara Brach from her book *Radical Acceptance* (2003), where body sensation is likened to the pulsating light of constellations in the sky, is especially fitting for eating disorders. The purpose of this body scan is to allow the children and adolescents to move away from a static view of their bodies to a more embodied awareness of present moment sensation. Brach says it best, "As I relaxed into feeling the sensations in my hands, I realized that there was no distinct boundary, no sense of defined shape . . . All I could perceive was the changing field of energy that felt like moving points of light in a night sky" (p. 99).

This mind-body focus on present moment body sensation is also the main way I target the second risk factor of *self-objectification*. Klein and Cook-Cottone (2013) write that self-objectification is the perception of oneself as an object rather than a subject. Adolescents with EDs will often complain about their appearance as if the way they look (or, more accurately, their perception of how they look) is the only valuable possession they have. Reminding an adolescent with an eating disorder of her accomplishments or good qualities usually backfires. However, when her attention is diverted to present moment sensation through the above mind-body yoga strategies, she is distracted from the objectifying and instead becomes more embodied and thereby naturally relates to her experience subjectively.

Another strategy I use to target this second risk factor of self-objectification is to ask participants to look through old issues of *Yoga Journal* after doing a shortened yoga sequence. Right after practicing yoga and before looking through the magazines, I ask adolescents to name how they feel different after practicing yoga than before. Some common answers are centered, relaxed, more confident or focused. I write these on a dry erase board in our yoga studio and then tell each participant to leaf through one of the magazines looking for an example of objectification (often in the advertisements) and an example of one of the good feelings listed on the board. The purpose of this exercise is to teach adolescents recovering from EDs how to practice discrimination as they transition from intensive treatment to their everyday lives. (I do NOT recommend this practice for children younger than 13 years of age, because they usually don't have the same issues with body image as adolescents do. As such, children may potentially be negatively influenced by magazine images that advertise the importance of body image.)

Drive for thinness, or the motivation to lose weight, is the third risk factor. Many experts agree this can be a motivating and/or maintaining factor in both anorexia and bulimia (Garner, 1991; Tylka, 2004; APA, 2015). One way this risk factor manifests in a yoga therapy group is participants' *body checking* or calorie burning behaviors. Body checking behavior refers to checking bony body parts such as wrists, collar bones or hips for perceived weight gain or loss. Calorie burning behaviors include shaking limbs while sitting or standing still in an effort to burn calories. Not only is it important for a yoga therapist to ask an adolescent engaging in such behaviors to stop for her own sake, but also for the sake of other adolescents patients who may be influenced by peer behavior.

The fourth risk factor is *body and emotional awareness*. Individuals who exhibit EDs practice such extreme eating and exercising behaviors that they lose touch with this awareness (Daubenmeier, 2005; Klein & Cook-Cottone, 2013). As a result, these patients not only show chronic fatigue and impaired hunger recognition, but impaired emotion recognition. The patients I see often genuinely don't know how they feel, because they've ignored feelings of all sorts for so long. This is in large part why I start yoga interventions for eating disorders by asking patients to simply notice body sensation. Even this can be challenging for an anorexic patient who has practiced starving herself for a long time. Such a patient benefits from group yoga practice by hearing peers who are further along in their treatment voice their awareness of physical sensations and emotional states with which she herself may have lost touch.

A possible fifth category of ED risk factors is childhood obesity. Lock and le Grange (2005) note that adolescents and older children who were obese at a younger age may suffer from poor body image. Many of these children and adolescents are subjected to a fair amount of bullying for not fitting into social norms. But the other insidious problem with childhood obesity leading to an eating disorder is the lack of recognition with regards to the eating disorder's onset. That is to say, a child may be well practiced in ED behaviors before it becomes noticeable that these behaviors are a problem.

Yoga may increase ED protective factors

Self-competence refers to one's sense of being capable or competent. As noted earlier, one of my individual patients Jarod said that yoga gave him his confidence back. In this way, the first and second protective factors are two facets of the same thing.

The third protective factor, *emotion regulation*, clearly follows after an individual recovers her body and emotional awareness. Emotion regulation refers specifically to one's ability to cope with negative emotions. The importance of this factor cannot be overstated, since it seems that those with eating disorders cope with negative affect through the ED and ED behaviors. An individual with an eating disorder will deal with difficult emotions by practicing ED behaviors, so learning strategies other than ED behaviors to regulate emotion in the face of difficult emotions appears key to recovery. Because of its emphasis on presentmoment body sensation, the yoga intervention "Body Sensations as Constellations" can help bolster the protective factor of emotion regulation. For example, when Jarod kept getting benched in baseball practice, he dealt with his disappointment by restricting his food intake and exercising excessively in his room at night. Through yoga, he learned to acknowledge negative feelings (like his worries about whether to go to college or not) by taking deep breaths and focusing on present moment body sensations in yoga poses.

Other pertinent research trends

Beyond the risk and protective factors, the Klein and Cook-Cottone review found three encouraging trends regarding ED treatment and yoga: Firstly, yoga seems to be safe with regards to ED and ED behaviors. In other words, those with eating disorders show no adverse effects from doing yoga. This is encouraging because there has been concern that yoga could cause patients with eating disorders to lose weight or otherwise become more fixated on ED behaviors. The studies in Klein and Cook-Cottone's review suggest that in fact, yoga is safe even for those with eating disorders. In particular, Carei and colleagues (2010) found that yoga treatment did not lower subjects' weight in their study.

Secondly, 40% of the 14 studies suggest that yoga practitioners are less likely to have an ED or ED behaviors. This might be interpreted to mean that doing yoga may bolster protective factors such as self-esteem and body awareness (Daubenmier, 2005; Dittmann & Freedman, 2009; Klein & Cook-Cottone, 2013). And third, most of the yoga interventions used in the studies were associated with fewer ED symptoms (Cook-Cottone et al., 2008; Scime & Cook-Cottone, 2008; McIver et al, 2009; Carei et al., 2010).

Several limitations were found with regards to the research reviewed by Klein and Cook-Cottone. The first is the absence of RCTs. In particular, the existing studies demonstrated significant weakness in research design. Also, many of these studies included primarily female subjects. While those with eating disorders are predominantly female, males *are* affected, and so not having male subjects represents a gap in our understanding of how yoga might help all those who suffer from eating disorders. Another limitation (even with the three RCTs included) was a lack of standardization of the yoga practice used. This means that not all subjects received exactly the same yoga sequence or treatment, which compromises to what extent the results can be generalized. A third limitation is the unaccounted-for influence of the yoga instructor, group dynamics within a particular class, and the variability of yoga instruction. As I mentioned in Chapter 2, individuals within a yoga group are often very influenced by the cohort of practitioners. A particularly supportive cohort may show better adherence and more positive results than one that is not.

Clearly, several steps need to be taken to show yoga's effectiveness for eating disorders. The most important step is to create an RCT with a standardized yoga protocol that can be replicated by others. Klein and Cook-Cottone offer additional suggestions:

"It is prudent to identify which factors influence the effectiveness of yoga interventions so that treatment can prescribed accordingly if yoga is to be considered an empirically supported adjunct therapy for EDs . . . (S)tudies comparing various dosages of the same form of yoga and investigations of different styles of yoga are needed to discern whether a particular type and/or dosage of yoga is associated with maximal ED-related benefits" (2013, p. 49).

Case studies

Though in a fledgling stage, current research suggests that yoga therapy may be an effective adjunctive therapy for treating eating disorders. My nine years of working weekly with children and adolescents suffering from eating disorders tells me that yoga therapy does in fact bolster protective factors and minimize risk factors. "Yoga offers a non-verbal, experiential adjunct to talking therapy that provides an opportunity for connection with the physical body and the inner experience" (Boudette, 2006, p. 170). While understanding current research is important, nothing is more powerful than reading the stories of those who have used yoga to help them in their treatment. Thus, three case studies follow to illustrate the power of yoga to address the mind-body nature of EDs, ED behavior, and body image issues.

Journaling to boost self-competence and emotion regulation

Sometimes the best interventions are the ones that a child or adolescent finds on her own. This past year, "Maria" (an 11-year-old girl on the eating disorder unit) was referred to me for individual yoga therapy. When I met with her to determine her goals for our sessions, Maria mentioned she liked to write. I asked her if she kept a journal and she said yes. I knew she would be leaving soon, so I suggested that she keep a log of her favorite poses. Maria took this task to heart, and brought back brightly colored pages filled with images and words (Figure 5.1).

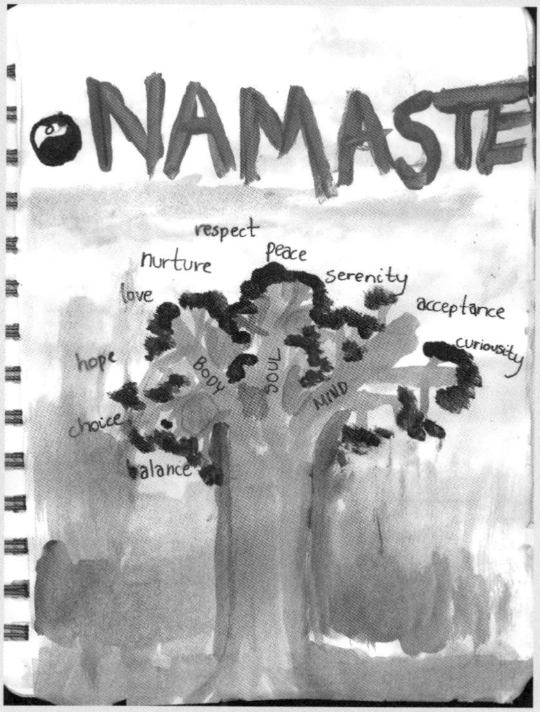

Figure 5.1
Maria's "Namasté Tree" symbolizes the positive states of mind she feels when she does yoga

Case studies *(Continued)*

Maria's pages show how she used her yoga practice to learn two important ED protective factors: emotion regulation and self-competence. Her illustration of "Namasté Tree" features many words indicating self-regulation like "serenity", "acceptance" and "peace." In addition, she used her journal to record the various individualized practices we created together. Figure 5.2 shows the morning practice we developed so that she could distract from the stress she felt right before eating breakfast. Maria demonstrated ownership of her yoga practice by color-coding each practice sequence.

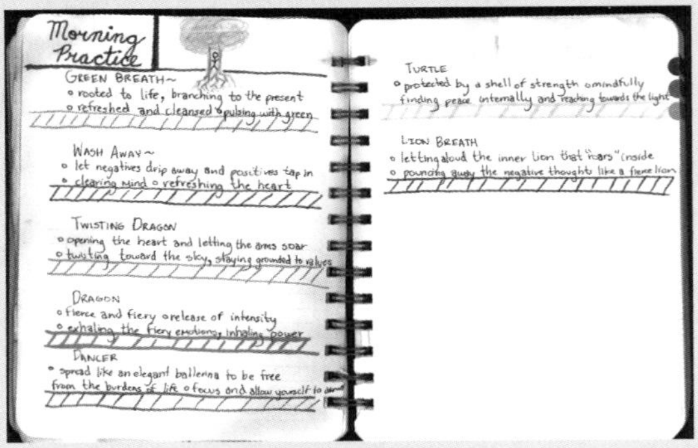

Figure 5.2
Maria's Morning Yoga Practice, designed to help distract and calm her

Andrea, an adolescent peer, heard about Maria's yoga "journaling" and requested individual yoga sessions to create the same kind of individualized home practice. She too demonstrated both self-competence and self-regulation in her journal pages as illustrated in Figure 5.3. She told me this page was important to her, because it reminded her of what she wanted to get from practice so that she didn't turn yoga into yet another form of exercise. This shows her increasing allegiance with self-regulation behavior over eating disordered behavior.

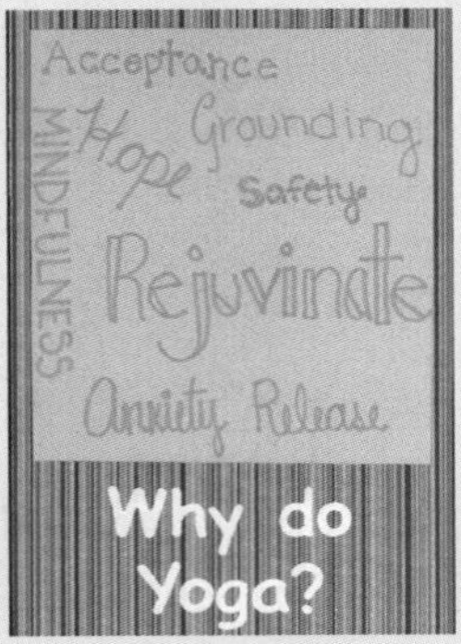

Figure 5.3
The first page of Andrea's yoga practice journal helped remind her of the healthy benefits of doing yoga, so she wouldn't turn it into exercise.

Case studies *(Continued)*

Jarod: The masculine perspective of eating disorders

Jarod, the 18-year-old male I mentioned earlier in this chapter, presented with a common disposition we see in boys with eating disorders. He reported being overweight as a child, but lost a lot of weight when he joined his junior high baseball team. When he started losing a lot of weight as a result of intensive practice, he received a lot of positive feedback. Though he loved to play, he said he was often benched. He remembers using the conditioning exercises he had learned to distract from the disappointment of not being allowed to play. This led to further dieting and exercising. After a while, he said he couldn't stop himself from compulsively engaging in exercise and dieting rituals.

Jarod was a leader among his peers when he was in treatment. When others in his ED cohort were stuck in body image issues and lack of motivation, Jarod knew what to say to motivate them. He started to see his positive influence on others. Because he received individual yoga therapy from me, I would often turn to him in yoga group, and ask him what yoga poses/interventions he thought might help the group. Interestingly, the most memorable yoga intervention we did together had nothing to do with poses: I invited Jarod to create a mandala on a yoga mat of all the things he loved, past, present and future to help him transition back into his life beyond high school and ED treatment.

He wrote in a good-bye letter to me, "(Yoga) has (shown) me that I can have a powerful effect on others. But most importantly (yoga) showed me how to find some happiness within myself" (personal communication, Summer 2012). His words echoed a 2009 Time magazine article on yoga therapy for mental health that said that yoga can "empower people while priming them to access their deepest emotions ("Psychotherapy Goes from Couch to Yoga Mat" by Alana B. Elias Kornfeld)."

In summary

Pediatric eating disorders are particularly complex for a number of reasons, including differences in children's versus adults' presenting symptoms, as well as the need for family involvement in a child's treatment. Yoga can be a wonderful adjunctive ED therapy, because it addresses the nonverbal, mind-body crisis of these disorders in a unique way. While research on the topic is sparse and not yet of a high quality, the results are promising and point to ways in which yoga research for pediatric EDs can be better studied.

One promising direction for yoga research for EDs would be to systematically study in an RCT how yoga may decrease ED risk factors and increase protective factors. Presented in this chapter are two types of yoga interventions that could be used in a study to explore yoga's effectiveness for EDs and body image issues.

Practice considerations

Here follow two yoga therapy interventions I have developed for eating disorder treatment for two different settings: I use the first asana sequence for adolescent patients with eating disorders; and I use the second intervention for multifamily group therapy since the family component is such an important aspect of treatment for children and adolescents with eating disorders. Refer to Chapter 9 for detailed instructions, modifications and contraindications of the poses.

Adolescents

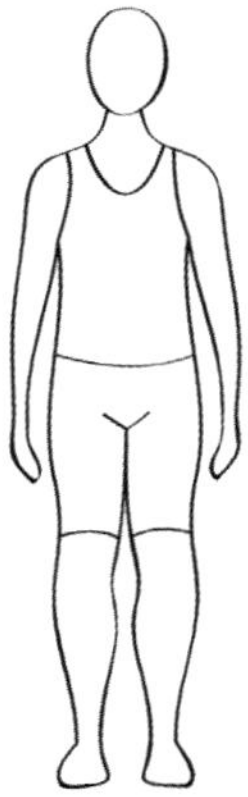

Figure 5.4
Tennis ball massage for feet

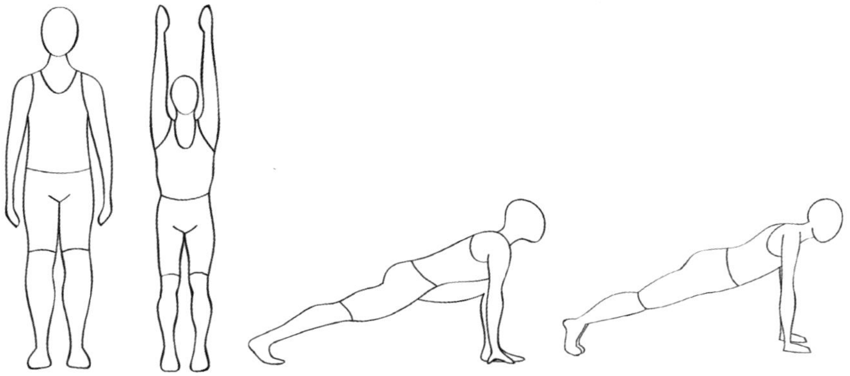

Figure 5.5
Surya Namaskar (Sun Salutation)—repeat this vinyasa once

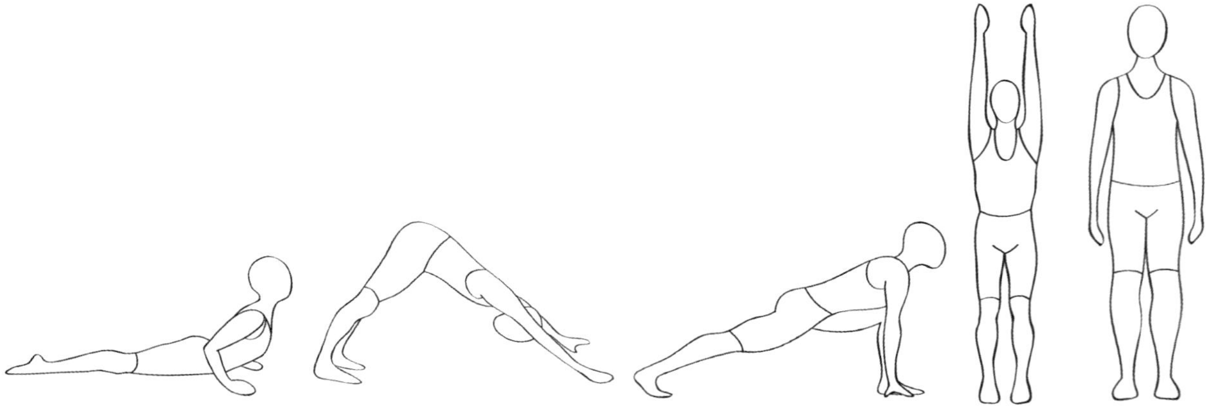

Figure 5.5 (continued)
Surya Namaskar (Sun Salutation)—repeat this vinyasa once

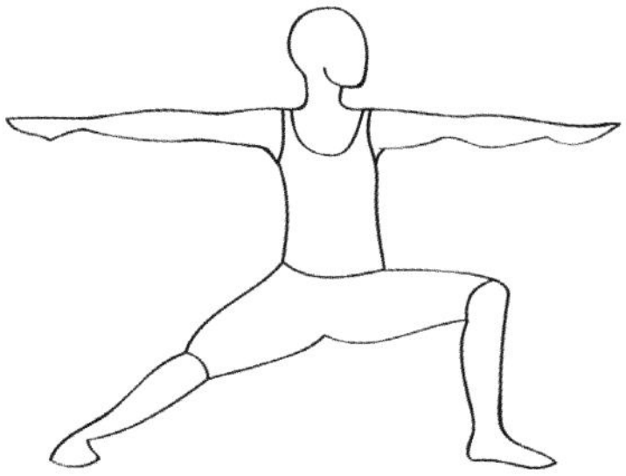

Figure 5.6
Virabhadrasana II (Warrior II)—repeat on both sides

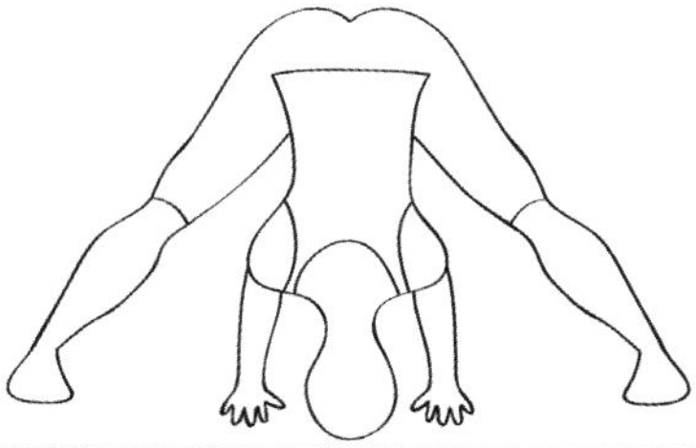

Figure 5.7
Prasarita Padottanasana A (Wide Legged Forward Fold)

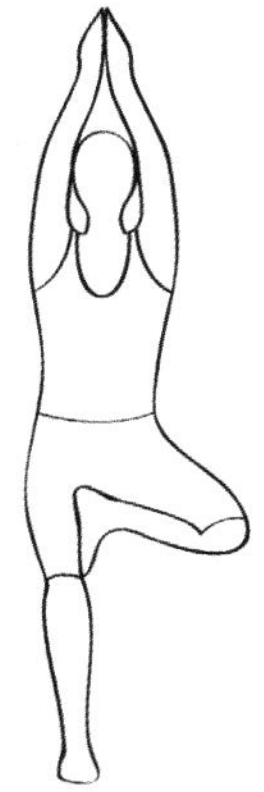

Figure 5.8
Vrksasana (Tree Pose)—repeat on both sides

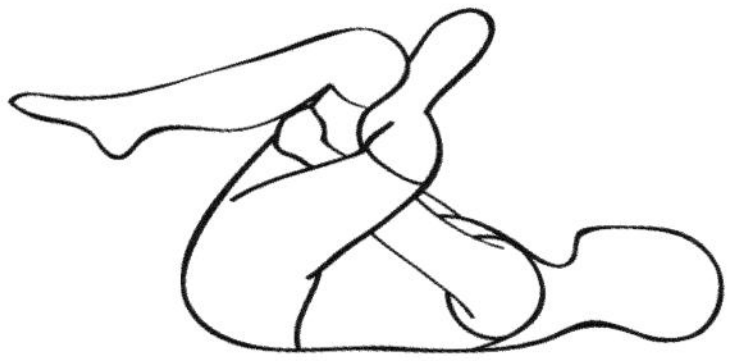

Figure 5.9
Sucirandhrasana (Eye of the Needle Pose)—repeat on both sides

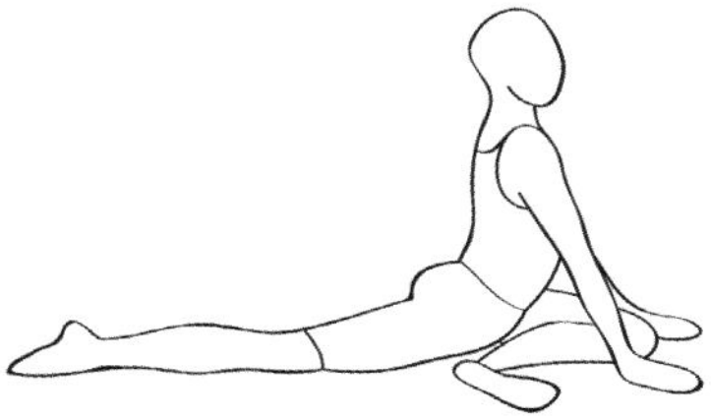

Figure 5.10
Eka Pada Rajakapotasana prep (Pigeon Pose)—repeat on both sides

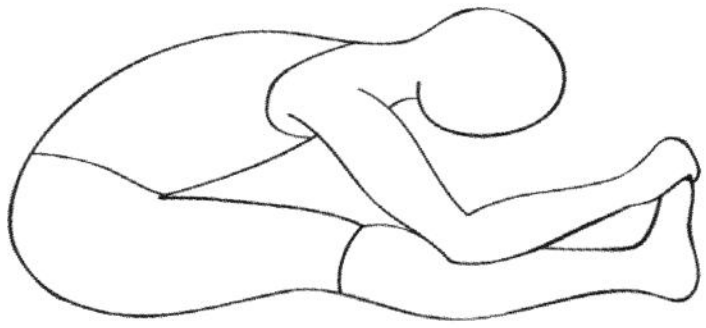

Figure 5.11
Paschimottanasana (Seated Forward Fold)

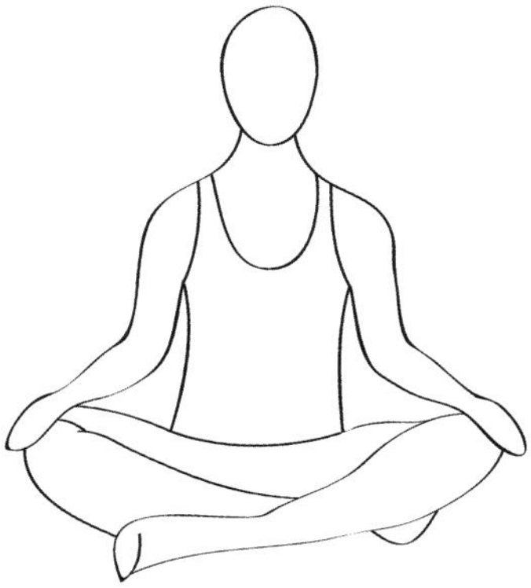

Figure 5.12
Sukhasana (Simple Sitting Pose) with Counting Breaths

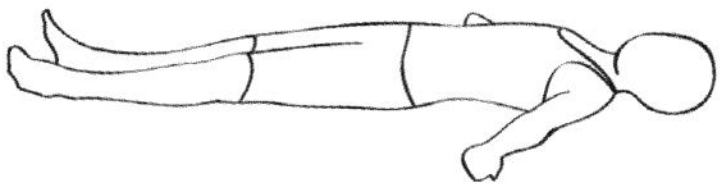

Figure 5.13
Savasana with Green Breath Visualization

Obstacle Course—cultivating empathy within the family system

The following intervention demonstrates how yoga therapy can be used as multifamily group therapy. The children and adolescent participants create an obstacle course from available objects (such as chairs, yoga mats, toys) that represent the obstacles of being in treatment for an eating disorder. For instance, almost all groups include an office chair that swivels to represent the disorientation of being in treatment and of the eating disorder itself. While the children create their unique obstacle course with the help of a staff facilitator, the parents meet in a separate room with other staff to talk about the fears they have about the obstacle course their children are creating. (It was during one of these parent groups that the father from the vignette likened his daughter's fear of brownies to his fear of heights.)

Once the patients complete the course, they explain the logistics of walking the obstacle course to the parent group. Many of the adolescent groups I have witnessed ask parents to close their eyes as they traverse the course to create a greater sense of disorientation. At this point in the intervention the patient group does not explain the symbolism behind the obstacles, since they are attempting to create a nonverbal, felt-sense of the eating disorder for their parents and families. The symbolism is saved for the end of the intervention, when parents talk about what the experience felt like to them, and their children discuss how the symbolism they intended ties in with the parents' felt experience.

The yoga therapy comes into play in how I ask the group to think about and discuss the dynamics and feelings that arise during the Obstacle Course. Participants are asked to practice *svadhayaya* (study of self) throughout the intervention. In the beginning, kids are asked to consider the question, "What are the obstacles in ED treatment?" In this way, they are taking an honest look at the ways in which they consciously or unconsciously resist treatment and getting better. Parents are asked to consider what fears arise as they imagine the obstacles their children might be creating for them. At the end, all participants share what the experience was like. In particular, parents are asked to share what thoughts, feelings and emotions arose as they did the obstacle course (which often mirrors the children's intended symbolism).

Child and parent groups are also asked to practice *satya* (or speaking the truth) in their own ways. The creation of the obstacle course itself is a way for children and adolescents to express difficult thoughts and feelings that they may be reticent to share in other overt ways. One of the "obstacles" that patients use a lot is asking their parents to write a hard truth about the eating disorder on a dry erase board.

Perhaps the most important yoga principle participants are asked to practice is *ahimsa* (non-violence) for themselves and their family members. Children are instructed to be compassionate with their parents while leading them through the obstacle course. Parents are encouraged to voice any concerns they have about doing the obstacle course after it is explained to them. But parents are also asked to express their concerns in "I feel" statements to maintain a non-questioning (and therefore non-aggressive) stance with their children.

Though I originally adapted this intervention from a kids' yoga game featured in Yoga Pretzels, it has become a rather intense experience, especially for parents. This has a lot to do with the creative input of the children and adolescents who take part in the Obstacle Course intervention. It is also one of the few practices in this book that does not include a single asana. This can be advantageous in allowing all members of the family to participate regardless of physical limitations. But the core reason for excluding asanas is simply that the intervention is a creative process among group members. Therefore, group members are free to include whatever tools they want to represent the obstacles of an eating disorder.

Suicidal Ideation and Non-Suicidal Self-Injurious Behaviors

6

Permission to feel: For several weeks I worked individually with "Stephanie," an adolescent girl who bounced around levels of psychiatric care for suicidal ideation and depression. She had not talked about her suicidality explicitly in our sessions, but her primary therapist had told me. Thus, when she was admitted for a third time, I decided to initiate a conversation about her suicidality so that we could include those feelings in her yoga treatment. She seemed angry and withdrawn when she entered the yoga room for our session.

"So, what brought you back to inpatient?" I asked nonchalantly.

"I had thoughts of killing myself," she replied, looking at the floor. "I'm glad right now that I didn't. But I don't know if or when the thoughts will come back, and that's really frustrating."

"Huh, it sounds really frustrating. You and I haven't talked about this before."

"I guess you're right. I'm not happy about these thoughts, they just show up."

She was still looking at the floor, her hair covering her face.

"Well, right now they're just thoughts. Obviously I wish you didn't have them. But as long as you do, the most important thing is that you talk about them, right?"

"Yeah, that's what my therapist says."

I noticed that Stephanie was talking about her thoughts of suicide, but still hadn't talked about the feelings underlying them. It seemed as though Stephanie was equating talking about her feelings (e.g. of sadness and depression) with the act of killing herself. She hadn't separated out her thoughts and feelings.

"What if you allow yourself to feel the feelings that bring up the desire to kill yourself, so that you can find out what you're feeling" I asked. "What if you give yourself permission to feel what you're feeling? That's what we practice in yoga, right?" Stephanie looked at me for a moment, and squinted.

"I hadn't thought about it that way, but I guess that's true—like, whatever feeling comes up I'm supposed to let it be."

Even though Stephanie had probably heard these very same ideas from her primary therapist, I knew that someone in as much pain as she was sometimes needs to hear the same point made in different ways by different people. I also knew that using the physical practice of yoga while mindfully allowing herself to feel might help Stephanie gain insight on a deeper level (Viggiano, 2014).

"Exactly!" I cheered. "You don't try to stop the feelings. Even if you're frustrated with trying to balance in Tree Pose, you go ahead and do it, because you know the more you practice the better you'll get. And it's going to end anyway."

Stephanie laughed. She looked me in the eye for the first time this session.

"Shall we do some yoga and check out how you're feeling?" I suggested

"Yeah, that sounds good," she said still laughing.

We practiced Tree Pose, as well as deep breathing. Stephanie had told me in the previous session that Tree Pose was one of her favorite poses, and we had just discussed the pose in relation to her feelings. But beyond her personal preferences, Tree Pose is an active pose. Viggiano (2014) says that action-oriented poses can empower an adolescent to feel like she is in

charge of her own experience. Stephanie said she felt calmer and more in control after the yoga session.
After that session Stephanie seemed more comfortable talking about her suicidal thoughts, which decreased the more she opened up to her treatment team. As a parting gift to me, she painted a canvas with a purple butterfly entitled "Yoga." Underneath the butterfly it reads "Validating, Safe, Heard, Calming and Accomplished." These are the things Stephanie said she felt when she was doing yoga.

First, empowering children and adolescents to identify and speak openly about the *feelings* (or the lack of feelings) that motivate their self-destructive actions is vital. Young people may not know what they are feeling. Thus, yoga therapy offers them a way to get in touch with what they're feeling—first, on the level of body sensation, and then on the level of felt experience and emotions.

Clearly, yoga therapy for acute symptoms like suicidal ideation and the like requires a yoga teacher or therapist to obtain appropriate training, experience and support. The key is for the yoga therapist to know the limits of her knowledge so that both client and therapist receive the support and guidance needed to make it a safe environment for all involved. Working within an integrated team of mental health professionals with expertise in acute symptoms of behavioral health is critical. At the Justice Resource Center, the yoga teachers all receive trauma-sensitive yoga training and adolescent patients attend yoga classes with a trauma therapist (Spinazzola et al., 2011). In my clinical practice at a pediatric hospital, I work with multidisciplinary teams and use their input to create integrated yoga therapy care plans for our shared patients.

Within such an integrated team model, yoga can be a wonderful therapy for both tolerating and distracting from negative feelings (van der Kolk, 2009; Spinazzola et al., 2011). Stephanie loved Tree Pose because she said it helped distract from her suicidal thoughts. But it also seemed to help her tolerate the feelings underlying her maladaptive thoughts. Much like the girl mentioned in Chapter 3 who suffered anxiety and did not like to fall out of Dancer Pose, Stephanie learned to tolerate falling out of Tree Pose. She learned that no one laughed at her or thought less of her.

This chapter explores how suicidal ideation (SI) and non-suicidal self-injurious (NSSI) behaviors differ from, as well as how they intersect, with each other. We will look at current models of therapeutic yoga for adults that can inform pediatric yoga therapy for these symptoms. An overview of yoga instructions and guidelines is presented for both SI and NSSI. Finally, specific sample practices are offered for adolescent populations.

Suicidal ideation and self-injurious behavior

Both suicidal ideation and self-injurious behaviors are symptoms of other affective issues (Woolery et al., 2004; Forbes et al., 2008; Walsh, 2012), such as depression and trauma covered in previous chapters. The acute symptoms of suicidal ideation and self-injury can lead to considerable consequences, such as persistent injuries to one's body, difficulties in using adaptive coping skills on a regular basis and death (Walsh, 2012). Suicidal ideation and self-injury can seem very similar to the untrained eye. Yet they may arise from very different contributing factors and issues, and have differing functions for individuals struggling with them. As such, it is important for a yoga therapist to understand these symptoms. While self-injury is extremely rare in school-aged and younger children, sadly, some school-aged children do experience suicidal ideation.

It is worth noting that the prevalence of self-injury has increased "markedly" (Walsh, 2012, p. 37). Walsh estimated that the rate of self-injury increased 250% over a 15-year period between 1980 and the late 1990s in the United States (going from 400 in 100,000 to 1,400 in 100,000). He speculates that this enormous increase could be due to both increased public awareness of the issue, as well as an increase in the number of people actually engaging in the behavior.

By contrast, the suicide rate in the U.S. is 11.5 in 100,000, which means an individual is 120 times more likely to self-injure than commit suicide. According to the Centers for Disease Control and Prevention (CDC, 2014), suicide is the third leading cause of death for youth between the ages of 10 and 24 years in the United States, or approximately 4,600 lives lost each year. In New Zealand, Fleming and colleagues (2007) found a gender difference in suicidal ideation among students ages 9 to 13 years. In a sample of 739 students, they found that 10.5% of females and 4.7% of males had made a suicide attempt within the last 12 months.

Walsh speculated a number of reasons for the increased prevalence of self-injury: environmental (such as school, an emphasis on competition, a lack of self-soothing skills, divorce/family strife, an overemphasis on physical appearance), direct media influence (music videos that show self-injury, or media celebrities who publicly discuss self-injuring, as well as videos of actual self-injury on internet sites like youtube.com), adolescent peer group, and internal psychological factors (such as mood dysregulation and trauma). Of concern is the fact that peer influence and media attention may cause an increase in prevalence in adolescents as well as younger and younger children to adopt these dysfunctional strategies.

Suicidality

Suicidal ideation is a common symptom of depression (Woolery et al., 2004; Forbes et al., 2008; Walsh, 2012). An individual who experiences suicidal ideation will do whatever it takes to stop the unwanted feelings (Walsh, 2012). In *Why People Die by Suicide* (2005), Thomas Joiner postulates three conditions necessary to complete a suicide:

1) Habituation (e.g. getting used) to pain
2) perceived burdensomeness and incompetence, and
3) thwarted belongingness.

The practice of self-injury is one way an individual can habituate to pain. Thus, we will explore the relationship between these two symptoms toward the end of this chapter. With regards to the second condition, suicidal individuals often see themselves as a burden on those they love and believe these loved ones would be better off without them. Lastly, individuals who consider suicide often feel a sense of isolation and a lack of belonging with their social group. Walsh notes that an individual who is suicidal is not as interested in destroying the physical body as he is with permanently ending aversive feelings.

Risk and protective factors

On its website, the American Foundation for Suicide Prevention (https://www.afsp.org/preventing-suicide/risk-factors-and-warning-signs, 2014) offers a list of both risk and protective factors. Risk factors include personal factors (such as a mental health diagnosis, own previous history of suicide attempts, a family history of suicide attempts or a serious medical condition), as well as environmental factors (such as a single high-stress event, a chronically stressful life situation, exposure to another person's suicide, and access to lethal methods of suicide). Protective factors include receiving effective mental health care, positive connections with family and friends, and effective emotion regulation skills.

Self-injurious behavior

In contrast, self-injurious behavior is an intentional, usually non-suicidal, behavior inflicted on one's body to relieve emotional suffering (Serani, 2012). For this reason, it is also known as non-suicidal self-injury (NSSI). NSSI may arise in those who experience *alexithymia* (the inability to identify emotions), mood dysregulation, and/or trauma (Herman, 1997; van der Kolk, 2009; Spinazzola et al., 2011; Serani, 2012; Walsh, 2012). Walsh (2012) distinguishes two categories of emotional suffering that motivate NSSI: experiencing too much emotion (such as anger, shame or guilt, anxiety/tension/panic, sadness, frustration or contempt) or experiencing too little emotion (often described by individuals as feeling "empty", or "zombie-like").

Risk and protective factors

Many experts say that the risk and protective factors for NSSI are similar to those of SI (CDC, 2014). However there are some important differences for clinicians, including yoga therapists, to be aware of when working with individuals who show symptoms of either.

What's the difference?

Psychiatrist Barent W. Walsh, PhD, who is the executive director of The Bridge of Central Massachusetts and a teaching associate in psychiatry at Harvard Medical School, lists 11 points of distinction between NSSI and SI in the second edition of his book *Treating Self-Injury: A Practical Guide* (2012). Along with the reasons for engaging in NSSI versus experiencing suicidal ideation, as described above, four additional features are important to consider when making a distinction between the two: *lethality, frequency, method* and *level of psychological pain*. Whereas NSSI are often low-lethality behaviors (e.g. the possibility of death is low), suicide attempts are usually high-lethality behaviors. Not surprisingly, this also affects the frequency of the two behaviors: NSSI is a high-frequency behavior with low lethality, whereas suicide is low-frequency behavior with high lethality. Here, suicide refers to completed suicides, not suicidal ideation.

The methods used by those engaging in self-injury tend to be quite different to those used by someone who is suicidal. Common methods of NSSI include cutting, burning, hitting, biting, pinching and carving. Indirect methods may also be used, such as substance abuse, eating disorders, risk taking (situational, physical and sexual), and medication discontinuation or abuse (Walsh, 2012). In contrast, relatively few methods are used in death by suicide. In the United States, the CDC (2014) reported that the top three methods used in suicides of young people include firearm (45%), suffocation (40%) and poisoning (8%).

Whether an individual is suicidal or engages in NSSI, she is experiencing some level of psychological pain (Walsh, 2012). The individual who is suicidal experiences on-going and excruciating psychological pain that fuels the "suicidal crisis" (Walsh, 2012, p. 13). On the other hand, the individual who engages in self-injury experiences intermittent psychological pain that is temporary. The self-injury itself relieves this mental anguish, if only temporarily.

The intersection of NSSI and suicidality

It may seem reassuring to learn that NSSI is not the same as suicide, and that self-injurious behaviors do not tend to result in death. But this is only part of the picture. NSSI may also lead to later suicidal behavior. Self-injury may be a way to habituate, or grow accustomed to, physical discomfort (Joiner, 2005; Walsh, 2012). Joiner (2005) says that deliberate acts of self-harm can desensitize an individual over time to the "monumental act" of killing oneself (Walsh, 2012, p. 22).

Yoga for acute symptoms

The best yoga treatments for children and adolescents suffering from SI and NSSI are those previously detailed in the chapters on trauma and mood dysregulation. In particular, the yoga intervention used at the Justice Resource Center and featured in Emerson and Hopper's book *Overcoming Trauma through Yoga* (2011) is an excellent option when working with acute symptoms. Erica Viggiano's yoga intervention called Mind Body Self Regulation Yoga® (patent pending: www.integrativelife.net) is also an excellent resource for adolescents experiencing behavioral symptoms of mood dysregulation. Viggiano herself has worked with adolescents suffering from SI and NSSI for many years, and therefore brings her experience with those populations to her trainings (personal communication, 17 July 2014).

Both SI and NSSI can arise from an individual's inability to regulate emotion, as well as one's reaction to life stressors. Yet the affective mechanisms causing SI and NSSI are somewhat different. Thus, the general guidelines for pediatric yoga therapy are also somewhat different.

Avoiding copycat behavior: Learning to identify and express the feelings that contribute to NSSI urges and suicidality is different to talking about the behaviors themselves, especially in a group setting. Because adolescents are particularly susceptible to mimicking peers' behavior, it is imperative to set very clear rules about not sharing NSSI or suicidal behavior when part of a group. Prinstein and colleagues (2010) found that "friends' self-harm was a significant predictor of NSSI above and beyond the effects of depressive symptoms" (p. 679). When establishing general group guidelines, it is helpful to differentiate among thoughts, feelings and behaviors. Sharing feelings is encouraged, but sharing self-destructive behaviors is unadvisable.

Yoga for suicidal ideation

To review, suicidality is often a symptom of major depression and/or trauma. Thus, the yoga techniques and practice recommended in this chapter mirror the principles of yoga for depression with some refinements. Several schools of yoga therapy recommend back-bending postures for symptoms of depression (Shapiro & Cline 2004; Woolery et al., 2004; Forbes et al., 2008). Forbes and colleagues (2008) assert that those who suffer from depression exhibit *hypotonicity* (low or weak muscle tone) in their bodies, which can lead to a slumped posture. Gentle backbends, such as a supported backbend over a roll, help reverse this trend in the body. While in a backbend, an individual may practice an uplifting breathing technique such as *viloma pranayama* with breath interruption on the exhalation. This particular version of *viloma pranayama* is used as a stimulating breathing practice by several yoga therapy programs (Iyengar, 1997; Kraftsow, 2002). McCall also recommends *viloma pranayama* with interruption on the exhalation for depression (2007).

Many of my adolescent patients who report suicidal ideation say they benefit from practices that help distract their minds from perseverating or racing thoughts of death and suicide. For this reason, mantra practice (especially when practiced aloud) can help move attention away from maladaptive, ruminative thinking. One particularly effective practice commonly used in Kundalini Yoga is the *Sa Ta Na Ma* mantra. Any practice (such as *Sa Ta Na Ma*) that orients an individual to the present moment can help "distract" from ruminative thinking (Lindenboim et al., 2007).

Suicide prevention training

Many individuals who experience suicidal ideation report feeling alienated by providers and caregivers who are surprised or ill-prepared to discuss acute symptoms of mood dysregulation, like suicidality (Sheean, 2010). As mentioned in Chapter 3, mood dysregulation often includes avoidance of unwanted thoughts and feelings that lead to dysfunctional changes in one's behavior. Some examples of these behaviors include panic attacks, dissociation, loss of control, or the desire and intent to kill oneself. Yet a yoga therapist may start working with an individual before knowing that the student is having thoughts of killing herself. As such, a yoga therapist working with individuals who experience acute mood dysregulation should seek training, as well as support from trained professionals, in suicide prevention.

A simple yet excellent training program for non-clinical community members is QPR, or *Question, Persuade and Refer* (QPR Institute website, 2011). The QPR Institute offers trainings for both classrooms and schools. Not only does QPR offer trainings for teachers and staff, but for youth peers as well, who may have more proximity and influence on their classmates and friends than adults.

Yoga for NSSI

Yoga for NSSI depends on the function the self-injurious behavior plays for an individual (i.e. is the adolescent self-injuring because of too much or too little emotion?). If an individual reports that she uses NSSI to reduce painful emotions, then a calming yoga practice is indicated. If she reports that self-injury helps her feel again (i.e. she feels empty or nothing) then a stimulating, yet grounding yoga practice is generally indicated. Using yoga practice in this way is known as *replacement behavior*, and is used frequently in DBT to help individuals replace problem behaviors (Linehan et al., 1999).

Either way, using a numerical scale to rate the intensity of sensation can help an individual gain a sense of empowerment and mastery in each pose. This is accomplished by asking the individual to rate the intensity of each pose using a subjective scale. For instance, I ask patients to rate the intensity of poses on a scale of 0–10, where 0 equals no intensity and 10 is maximum intensity. Once an individual has warmed up with a few yoga poses, I ask him to modify the pose until the level of intensity is between 5 and 7. This empowers the individual to decide for himself whether he should go deeper into the pose, or back out of it a bit. In addition, he learns how to increase intensity of sensation in a no-violent, mindful way. Anecdotally, clients have shared with me that this helps them learn to regulate physical sensation, which in turn seems to help them regulate emotions as well.

Further yoga training for acute behavioral health issues

To better understand the emotional landscape in which SI and NSSI arise, it is helpful for a yoga therapist to take specialized training in yoga for mental health. Two excellent yoga training programs for behavioral health are Amy Weintraub's LifeForce Yoga® for depressive symptoms and Bo Forbes' Integrative Yoga Therapeutics® for mood dysregulation. Both training programs have been researched (Bennett et al., 2008; Forbes et al., 2008), and Forbes draws upon her experience and training as a psychologist as well as a yoga therapist. Though both programs are geared toward adult clientele, a yoga therapist or teacher who is accustomed to working with children and adolescents could conceivably adjust these methods for younger populations.

In summary

Both suicidal ideation and self-injury are symptoms of more global mood dysregulation. This dysregulation may be a function of the emotional challenges of normal adolescence, or other more serious etiology such as anxiety, depression or trauma. Though school-aged and younger children rarely report self-injury, some do report suicidal ideation. It is important to take such reports seriously, and to listen with compassion and non-judgment. In addition, the increased prevalence of adolescent self-injury raises the question of whether we need to also be on the look-out for signs of NSSI in younger children.

Before working with children and adolescents with acute mood dysregulation, it is important for a pediatric yoga therapist or teacher to receive specialized training in SI and NSSI. Pediatric yoga therapists working in behavioral health should work closely with an integrated team of behavioral health professionals as well as receive specialized training in suicide prevention and self-injury. Such training and collaboration will help the yoga therapist to develop an informed and effective yoga therapy regimen for acute symptoms such as SI and NSSI.

Practice considerations

Adolescents with SI

This sequence includes several standing poses, which are meant to be grounding and help the practitioner focus on body sensation versus suicidal ideation or other negative ruminations. However, if the amount of standing poses is dysregulating for an individual, listen to your instincts as a teacher/therapist and defer to the individual's needs. Refer to Chapter 9 for detailed instructions, modifications and contraindications of the poses.

Ring a bell to indicate the beginning of the yoga therapy session.

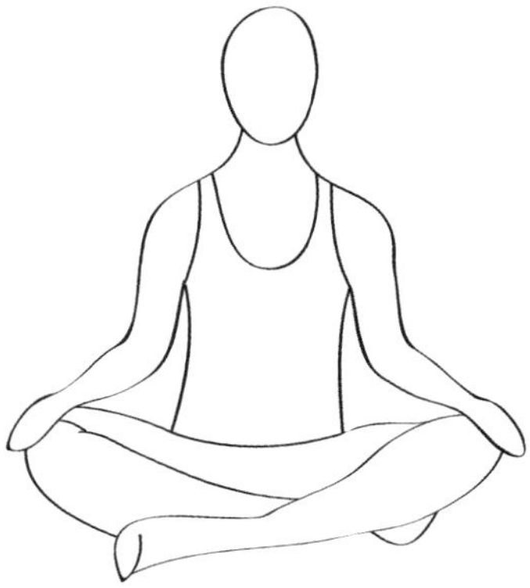

Figure 6.1
Sukhasana (Simple Sitting Pose) with Snake Breath

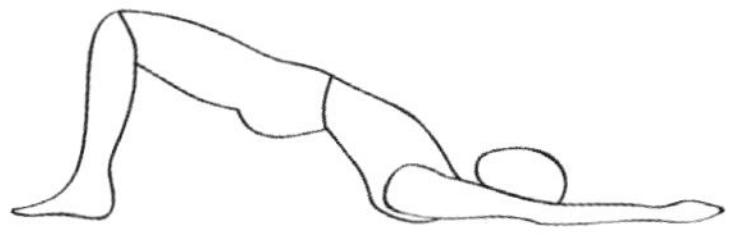

Figure 6.2
Bridge Pose Vinyasa—repeat five times

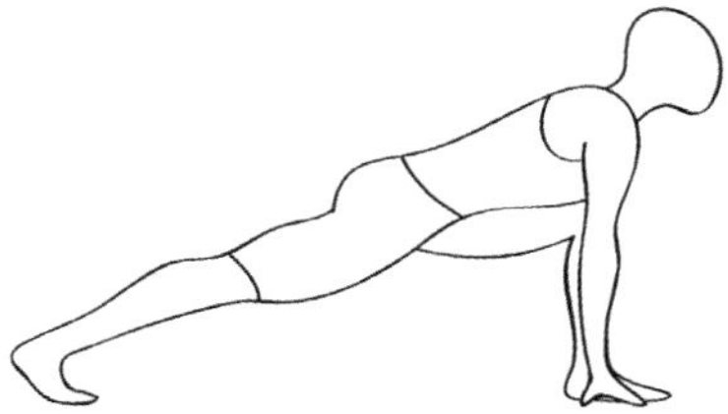

Figure 6.3
Lunge—repeat on both sides

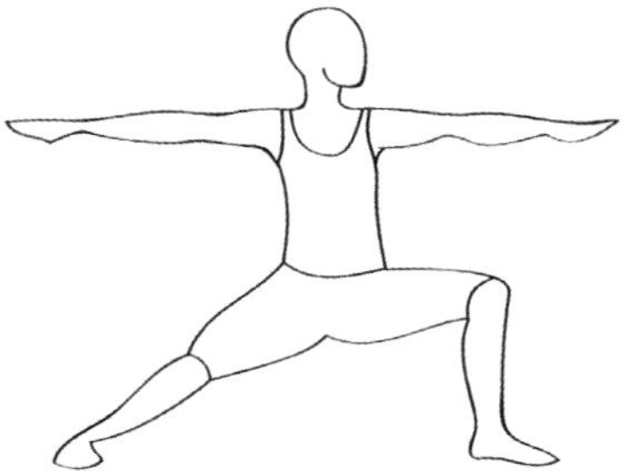

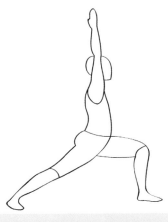

Figure 6.4
Virabhadrasana II (Warrior II)—repeat on both sides

Figure 6.5
Virabhadrasana I (Warrior I)—repeat on both sides

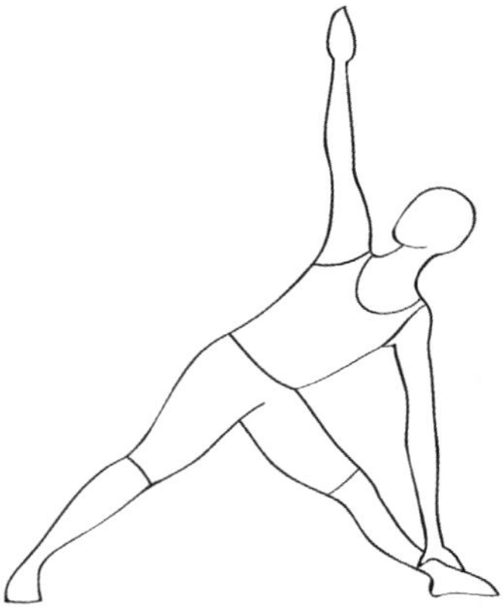

Figure 6.6
Utthita Trikonasana (Triangle)—repeat on both sides

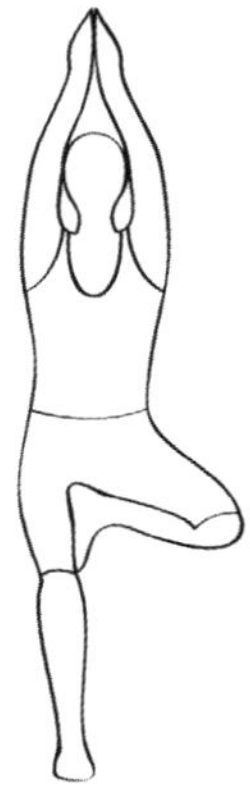

Figure 6.7
Vrksasana (Tree Pose)—repeat on both sides

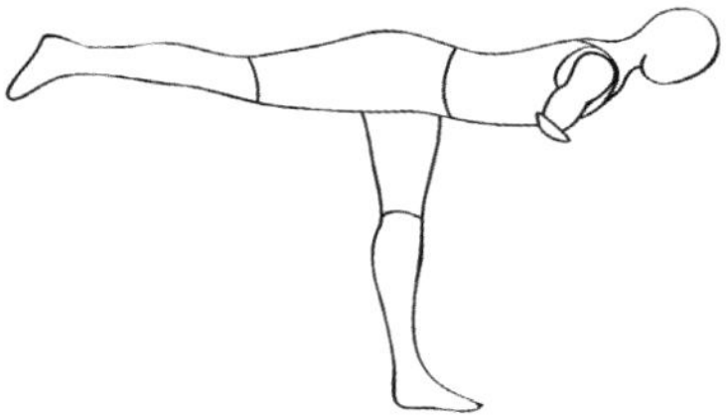

Figure 6.8
Dikasana B (Airplane Pose)—repeat on both sides

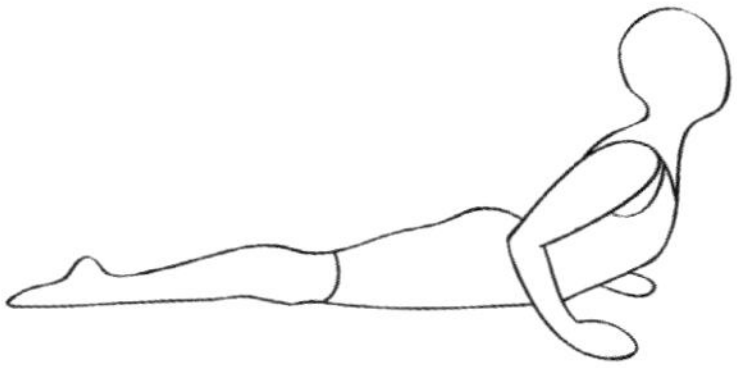

Figure 6.9
Bhujangasana (Cobra)

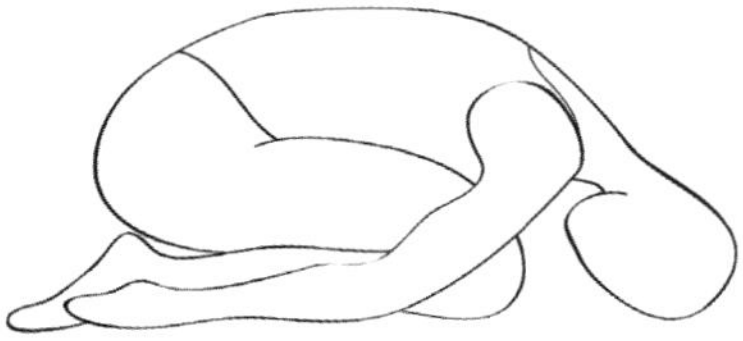

Figure 6.10
Balasana (Child's Pose)

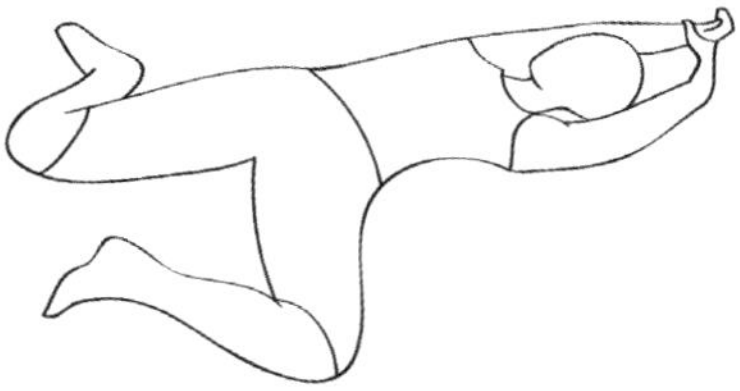

Figure 6.11
Windshield wipers

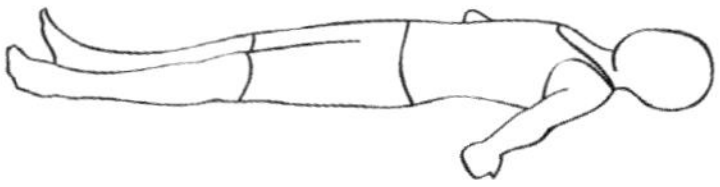

Figure 6.12
Savasana with short Yoga Nidra (5–10 minutes)

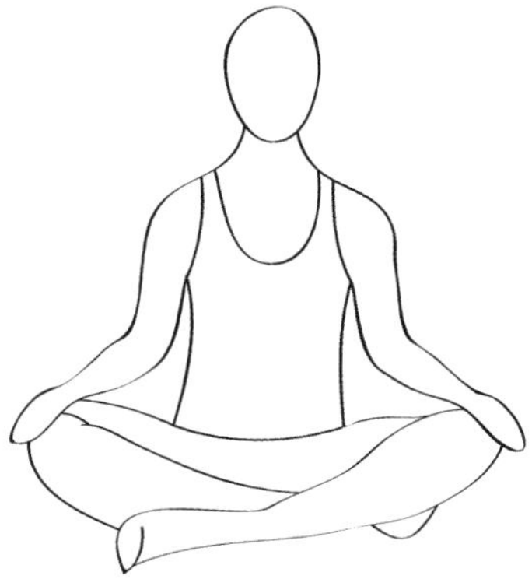

Figure 6.13
Sukhasana (Simple Sitting Pose) with Counting Breaths

Adolescents with NSSI

This sequence includes several standing poses, which are meant to be grounding and focusing to distract attention away from or replace the desire to self-injure. However, if the amount of standing poses (or sun salutations) is dysregulating for an individual, listen to your instincts as a teacher/therapist and defer to the individual's needs.

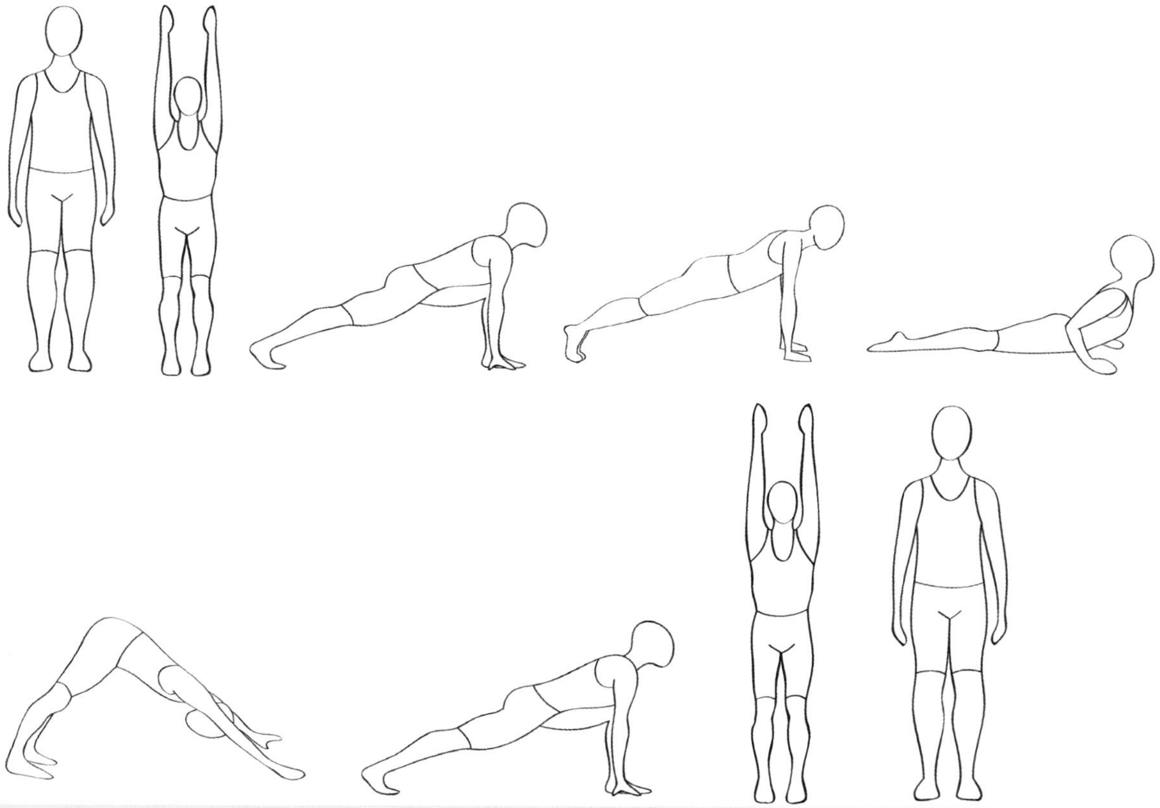

Figure 6.14
Surya Namaskar (Sun Salutation)—repeat this vinyasa three times

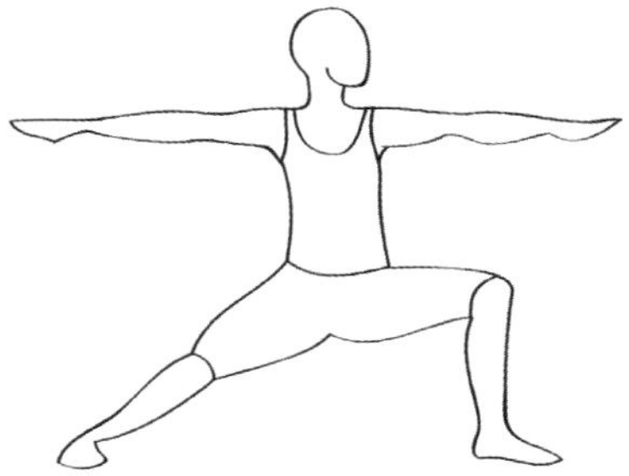

Figure 6.15
Virabhadrasana II (Warrior II)—repeat on both sides

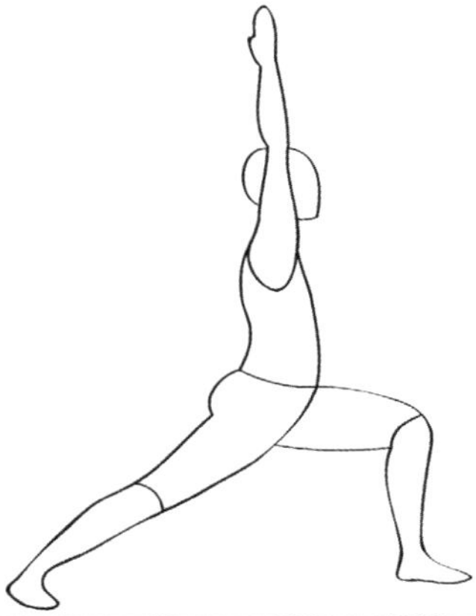

Figure 6.16
Virabhadrasana I (Warrior I)—repeat on both sides

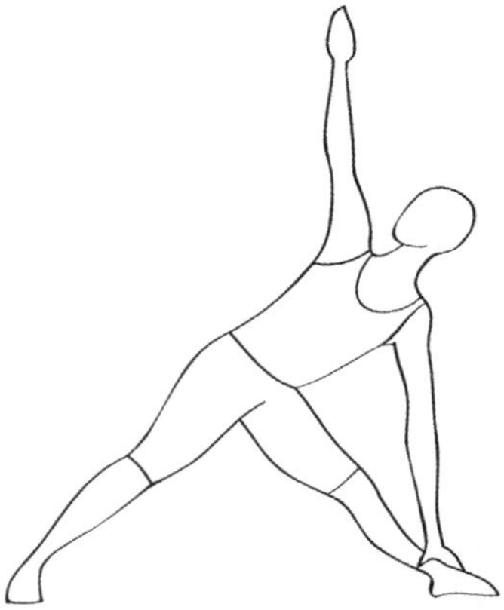

Figure 6.17
Utthita Trikonasana (Triangle)—repeat on both sides

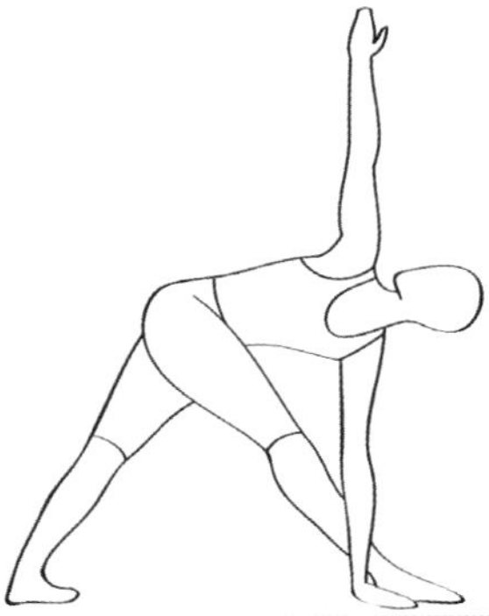

Figure 6.18
Parivrtta Trikonasana (Reverse Triangle)—repeat on both sides

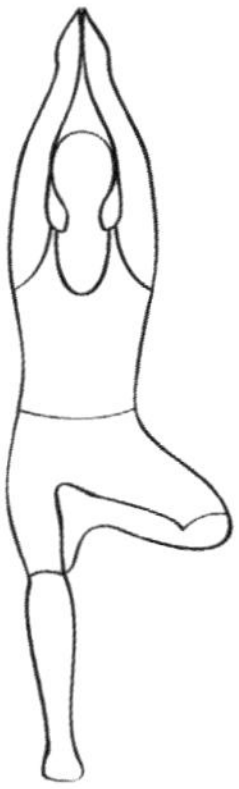

Figure 6.19
Vrksasana (Tree Pose)—repeat on both sides

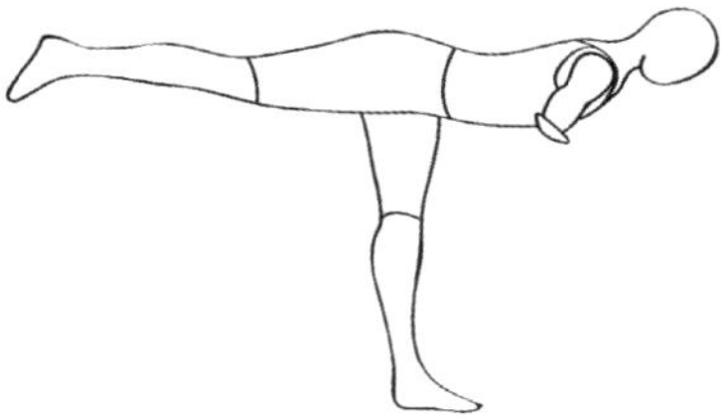

Figure 6.20
Dikasana B (Airplane Pose)—repeat on both sides

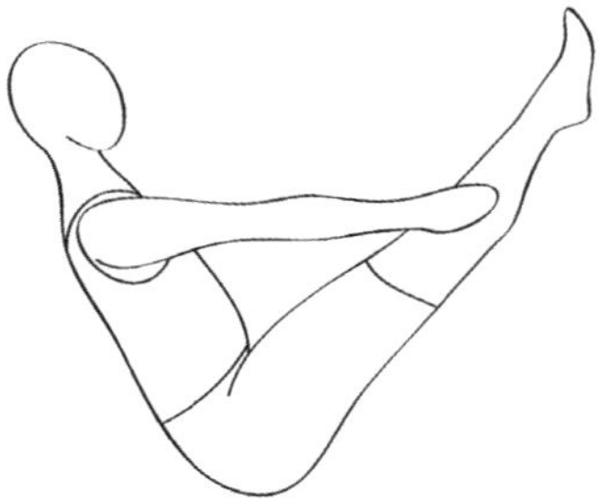

Figure 6.21
Paripurna Navasana (Boat Pose)

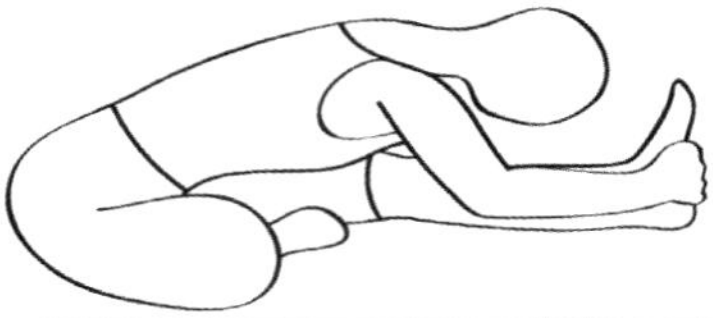

Figure 6.22
Janu Sirsasana (Runner's Stretch Pose)—repeat on both sides

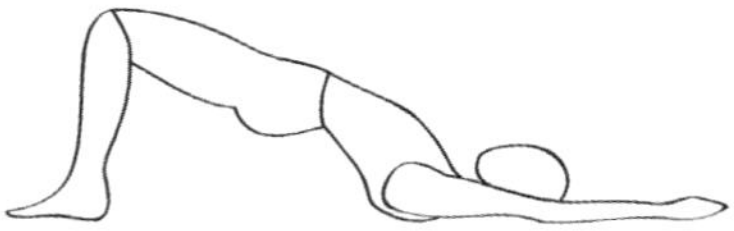

Figure 6.23
Setu Bandha Sarvangasana (Bridge Pose) Vinyasa—repeat five times

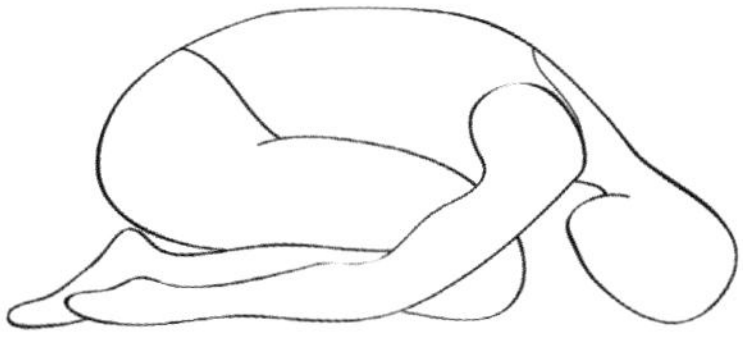

Figure 6.24
Balasana (Child's Pose)

Yoga Nidra (if little to no trauma) or Sa Ta Na Ma mantra (if moderate to severe trauma/hypervigilance).

Psychosis

7

A boy came to my psychiatric day treatment yoga group and shared that he had auditory and visual hallucinations that made it hard for him to focus. During the session I noticed his motor movements had slowed, and he was staring off into space. It looked as if his internal world of hallucinations had distracted him from asana practice. I asked if he'd like some help, and though it took him a moment to respond, he said yes. As I physically assisted him to bend and straighten his leg in a supine stretch, I noticed that his muscle movements become smoother with each repetition. In addition, his eyes lost their far off look and he reported being more oriented to the present moment.

Like this boy in my day treatment yoga group, children and adolescents who are in the midst of psychosis often have a distant look in their eyes, and have a hard time moving their bodies at will. When stressed, their minds tend to play tricks on them (Henry, 2013). Yet there is misunderstanding in the media and a lack of clarity in the mental health field of what exactly psychosis is.

The myths and mystery of psychosis

In the media, psychosis is often conflated with other serious mental health issues. One blogger from the United Kingdom (UK), "Henry" put it well: "People can be scared by the word 'psychosis.' It turns out that using that word, thanks to the media, tends to make people think you're a serial killer" (Henry, 2013). However, individuals who suffer from psychosis are not serial killers, and are not routinely violent. In a review article for the *Canadian Journal of Psychiatry*, Pamela Taylor (2008) wrote, "Public fears about individuals with psychotic illnesses are largely unfounded" (p. 647). In fact, individuals who suffer from mental illness, including psychosis, are more likely to be victims of violence than perpetrators (Hiday et al., 1999; Stuart, 2003). Taylor (2008) concedes that psychosis may "raise the risk" of an individual being violent, but that 95–99% of violence in society is not due to mental illness. In a review for the journal *World Psychiatry*, Heather Stuart (2003) found that socio-demographic and socio-economic status, as well as substance abuse issues, are greater determinants of violent behavior than mental illness.

Most importantly, psychosis is not the same as *psychopathy*. Psychosis is a symptom. Psychopathy is a personality disorder characterized by lack of remorse and cold, calculating behavior. Ted Bundy was a psychopath. In contrast, John Nash the Nobel Laureate in Economics whose life story was featured in the film *A Beautiful Mind*, exhibited psychotic behavior.

In the field of mental health, a clear understanding of psychosis, and its close companion schizophrenia, is still evolving. "While the diagnostic features of schizophrenia have remained unchanged for more than 100 years, the mechanism of illness has remained elusive" (Heckers et al., 2013, p. 11). What is clear is that psychosis is in a group of mental health issues that rank among the most severe (Bangalore & Varambally, 2012; Heckers et al., 2013). Treatment usually involves a good deal of antipsychotic medications, which are expensive and deliver suboptimal results (Duraiswamy et al., 2007; Bangalore & Varambally, 2012). In addition, up to 50% of patients with a first episode of psychosis suffer from long-term issues with psychosis (Huber et al., 2008).

Finally, many of the current antipsychotic drugs cause major physical health problems such as obesity and diabetes Bangalore & Varambally, 2012).

Yoga therapy may offer an adjunctive solution to this dilemma. Three articles on yoga for psychosis or schizophrenia (one RCT regarding yoga for schizophrenia, and two meta-analyses on yoga for schizophrenia or yoga for major psychiatric diagnoses) found that yoga appears to be a cost-effective, low-risk and viable long-term adjunctive treatment for these issues (Duraiswamy et al., 2007; Cabral et al., 2011; Bangalore & Varambally, 2012). But before delving into the benefits of yoga for psychosis, let's explore what psychosis is.

Psychosis

Psychosis is a loss of contact with consensus reality that includes *delusions* (false beliefs about one's identity or what is happening) and *hallucinations* (either seeing or hearing things that aren't there). Broome and colleagues (2005) report that risk factors for psychosis include genetics (either hereditary or developmental damage resulting in dopamine deregulation), substance abuse (such as amphetamines or cannabis), social adversity (such as migration or social isolation), or behavior changes that alter an individual's perception of reality (such as isolating oneself from friends and family).

The UK blogger Henry who created the video "Psychosis Isn't Anything Like a Badger" points out that someone who is susceptible to psychosis will often become psychotic during times of great stress (Henry, 2013). I worked with a 16-year-old girl who had a psychotic break after a series of life stressors, including an out-of-state move, the death of a beloved family member, and challenges fitting in at school. She struggled with voices that told her that members in her family were devils, or that she herself was a devil.

Early warning signs

If a young child reports hallucinations, assessment and treatment should be sought immediately. The reasons for a child's hallucinations could be neurological problems, bipolar disorder, or childhood schizophrenia—a very rare, but real, phenomenon. However, it is more likely for adolescents and young adults to report first episode psychosis that leads to a diagnosis like schizophrenia or bipolar (National Association of Mental Health, 2014).

The National Alliance on Mental Illness (NAMI) lists the early warning signs of psychosis on its website:

- Sudden drop in grades
- New trouble thinking clearly or concentrating
- Suspiciousness/uneasiness with others
- Decline in self-care or personal hygiene
- Spending a lot more time alone than usual
- Increased sensitivity to sights or sounds
- Mistaking noises for voices
- Unusual or overly intense new ideas
- Strange new feelings or having no feelings at all

Associated diagnoses and symptoms

Though psychosis is often associated with the DSM-V diagnosis of schizophrenia, psychosis is not solely a symptom of schizophrenia (Heckers et al., 2013). The confusion is understandable, though, because psychosis is *the* defining feature of schizophrenia.

Psychotic features are also present in various forms of bipolar and mixed affective disorders (National Institute of Mental Health, 2014? Ostergaard et al., 2013). Due to the complexity of these presentations, we will not go into detail about them. However, it is helpful to understand another symptom that is often associated with psychosis—*mania*. Mania is a defining symptom of bipolar I, and is characterized by excessive energy and abnormally high arousal or mood. During a manic cycle, individuals often need less sleep, may have delusions of grandeur, and may exhibit increased creativity and/or productivity. In more extreme cases, this manic state leads to psychotic symptoms like hallucinations and delusions (Cherry, 2014).

Yoga for psychosis

Yoga appears to offer the following benefits for those who suffer from psychosis:

1) a reduction of psychotic symptoms and depression
2) improved cognition
3) reduction in stress
4) increased physical health, and
5) positive neurobiological changes

(Duraiswamy et al., 2007;Bangalore & Varambally, 2012). Firstly, in what Duraiswamy and colleagues (2007) report is the first randomized control trial on the benefits of yoga for schizophrenia, they found promising results regarding a reduction of psychotic symptoms and depression for 41 subjects who suffer from schizophrenia. However, Duraiswamy, Bangalore and their colleagues note that more research needs to be done to determine the mechanism by which yoga relieves these symptoms. Secondly, yoga seems to improve cognitive functioning. My young patients with psychotic features tell me that yoga helps them orient to consensus reality, and this seems to keep hallucinations and delusions at bay. Thirdly, yoga reduces stress, which could potentially reduce or diminish one's psychotic symptoms (Duraiswamy et al., 2007). Relatedly, yoga may improve an individual's physical health—the fourth potential benefit of yoga for psychosis. As Duraiswamy and colleagues (2007) point out, "regular physical exercise also mitigates the effects of stress" (p. 230). This is turn may help individuals reduce the number of antipsychotic medications that can cause obesity, diabetes and other health issues (Duraiswamy et al., 2007; Bangalore & Varambally, 2012). Fifthly, Bangalore and colleagues (2012) propose that yoga may increase an individual's quality of life through neurobiological changes, such as an increase in oxytocin levels.

In practice, I follow four principles for creating effective yoga treatments for children and adolescents suffering from psychosis that relate to the aforementioned potential benefits. Firstly, "action-oriented" techniques, as Viggiano (2014) calls them, help individuals focus cognitively and stay oriented to the here and now. Action-oriented practices are of two types: activating and calming. For instance, sun salutations and challenging arm or standing balance poses are action-oriented poses that activate the nervous system. Repeating the *Sa Ta Na Ma* mantra while touching the fingers to thumb is an example of an action-oriented practice that calms the nervous system. Secondly, interventions that orient the individual to his environment are helpful, such as focusing on the five senses while doing yoga poses. Thirly, practices that engage the individual in social interaction are helpful. For instance, if a number of adolescents tell me they experience psychosis I will lead the group in a mildly energizing practice, in which I encourage conversation about what participants are feeling in the poses. Participants are encouraged to share what alignment strategies work for them to make the pose easier or feel better. This not only creates social bonding but also orients the participants to their social environment. Finally, I tell participants to stop doing the technique any time they feel strain or irritation that does not immediately subside with the breath or relaxing into the practice.

Contraindications for psychosis

One size does not fit all

A letter to the editor featured in the November 2007 issue of the *American Journal of Psychiatry* reported potentially negative effects of intense yoga practice for psychosis. After 10 years of being symptom-free, a man with a history of drug-induced psychosis attended a Bikram yoga teacher training, and exhibited psychotic behavior while in the training. The psychiatrists who authored the letter, Drs. Jessica Lu and Joseph Pierre, concluded that "(I)ntensive yoga and meditation have been reported in association with altered perceptions and full-blown psychotic episodes" (p. 1761).

The sentiment in the above letter reflects a growing understanding in the extant yoga research with regards to mental health and yoga: Different yoga techniques create different effects in the mind and body (Cabral et al., 2011). Yoga Master B.K.S. Iyengar cautioned that choosing poses that aren't appropriate for an individual's condition may "adversely affect his or her health" (2001, p. 238). In particular, meditation (Booth, 2014) and rigorous yoga practices (Lu & Pierre, 2007) are contraindicated for those who experience psychosis, or other acute symptoms of mental illness. A *contraindication* is anything (drug, technique, or other method) that may cause more harm than benefit.

The Guardian tackled the issue of meditation and mental health in an online article by Robert Booth. In the article Booth (2014) cites Marie Johansson, clinical lead at Oxford University's Oxford Mindfulness Centre, who emphasized the mental rigor required in meditation practices and retreats. Meditation generally requires one to pay attention to the contents of one's thoughts without getting lost in the thoughts. This is not possible for people with psychosis, or other highly disturbed states of mind, because they are literally deluded by their thoughts. Thus, Johansson points out that meditation can be a very disempowering experience for those with mental instability (Booth, 2014).

While no research could be found to validate the claim that rigorous yoga practices are contraindicated for psychosis, my experience as a clinician working with psychosis leads me to agree with it. In the same way that meditation can cause mental stress, rigorous yoga poses can cause physical stress. If an individual cannot breathe deeply in an intense yoga pose, she may experience panic or other symptoms of acute stress. A common mistake of beginners to both meditation and yoga is not to breathe or relax into the intensity of the experience. When one does not relax, the experience is intense and aversive—in other words, it becomes a stressor rather than an outlet for stress. As a result, it is important to keep an on-going dialogue with individuals who are prone to psychosis while practicing yoga.

In summary

Psychosis is a symptom that occurs in two of the most severe and disabling mental health diagnoses—schizophrenia and bipolar I. Treatment-as-usual includes antipsychotic medications, which are expensive and deliver sub-optimal results. Unfortunately up to 50% of patients with a first episode of psychosis suffer from long-term mental health issues. In addition, many of the current antipsychotic drugs cause major physical health problems such as obesity and diabetes.

Yoga appears to be a cost-effective, low-risk and viable long-term adjunctive treatment for these issues. Studies show that yoga may be beneficial for psychosis in the five following areas:

1 a reduction of psychotic symptoms and depression
2 improved cognition

3 reduction in stress
4 increased physical health
5 positive neurobiological changes.

This writer has found four effective strategies when using yoga as an adjunctive treatment for psychotic features:

1 use action-oriented poses that either mildly activate or calm the nervous system
2 use interventions that orient the individual to his environment
3 use practices that engage the individual in social interaction
4 encourage students to stop any technique that causes strain or irritation that could trigger psychotic thoughts or behavior.

As helpful as yoga appears to be for psychotic features, meditation and rigorous yoga practices are contraindicated. Meditation may actually exacerbate psychotic thinking through silence and rigorous mental effort. Challenging yoga poses may overstimulate the nervous system and lead to psychotic thinking and behavior.

More research needs to be done regarding the mechanisms by which yoga is beneficial to psychosis. However, a well-informed yoga therapist or teacher who knows the signs to look for and has the support of a treatment team, may offer a much-needed and effective adjunctive treatment to those who suffer from psychosis. Refer to Chapter 9 for detailed instructions, modifications and contraindications of the poses.

Practice considerations

Adolescents

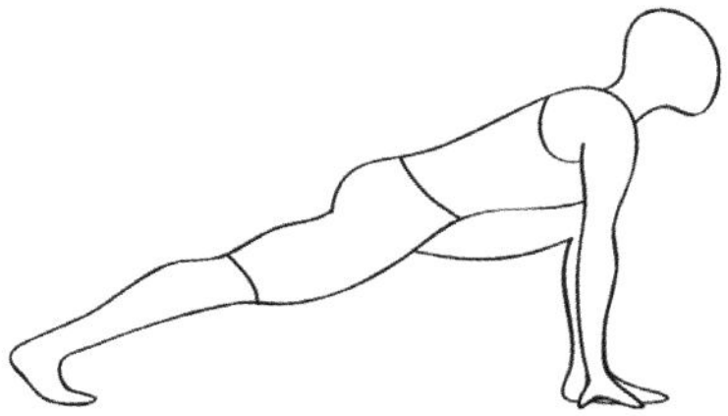

Figure 7.1
Lunge—repeat on both sides

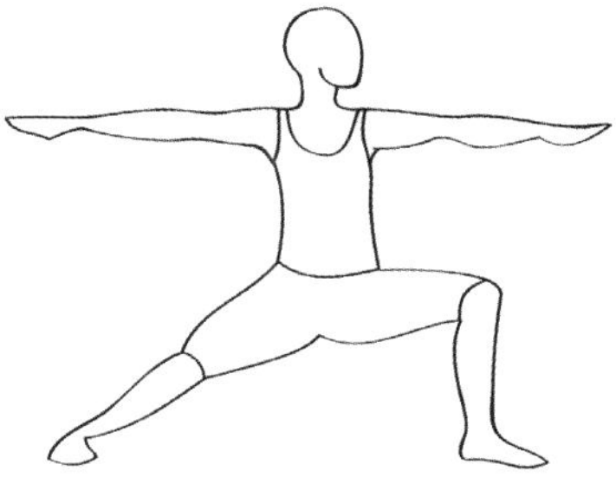

Figure 7.2
Virabhadrasana II (Warrior II)—repeat on both sides

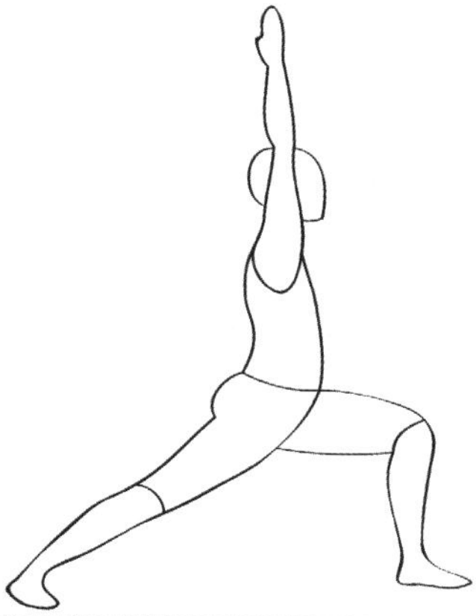

Figure 7.3
Virabhadrasana I (Warrior I)—repeat on both sides

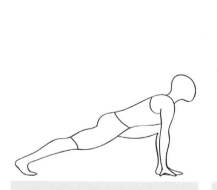

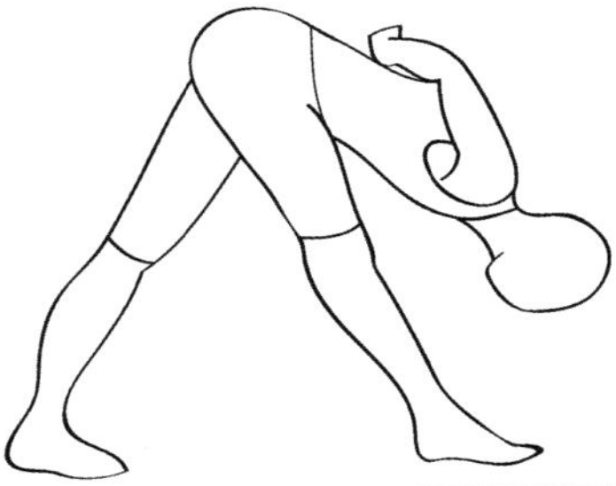

Figure 7.4
Parsvottanasana (Pyramid Pose)—repeat on both sides

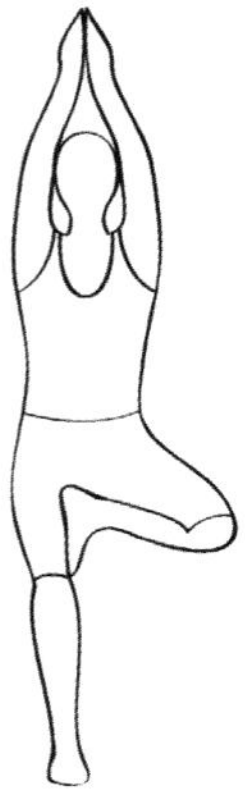

Figure 7.5
Vrksasana (Tree Pose)—repeat on both sides

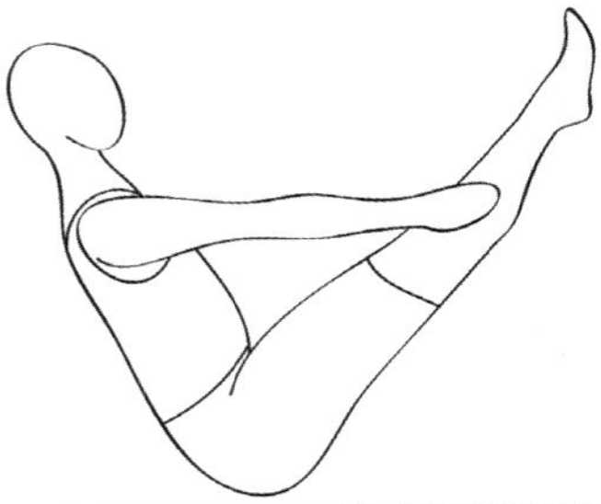

Figure 7.6
Paripurna Navasana (Boat Pose)

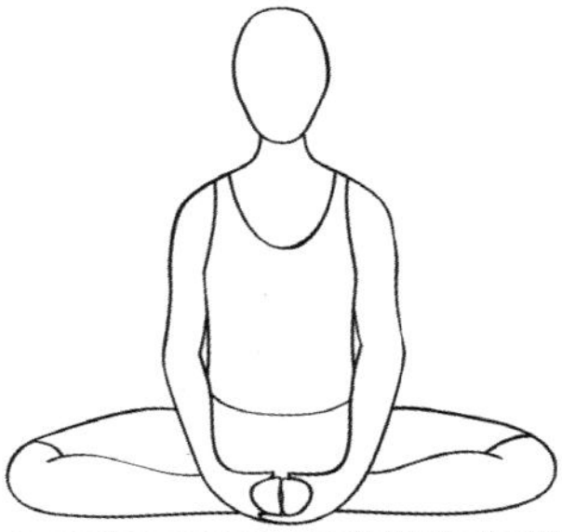

Figure 7.7
Baddha Konasana A (Cobbler's Pose)

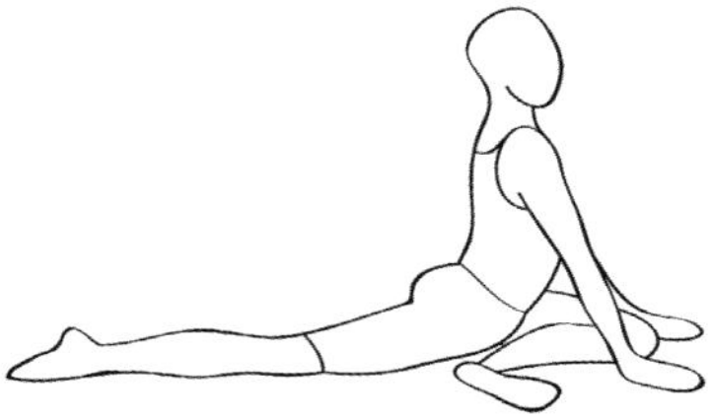

Figure 7.8
Eka Pada Rajakapotasana prep (Pigeon Pose)—repeat on both sides

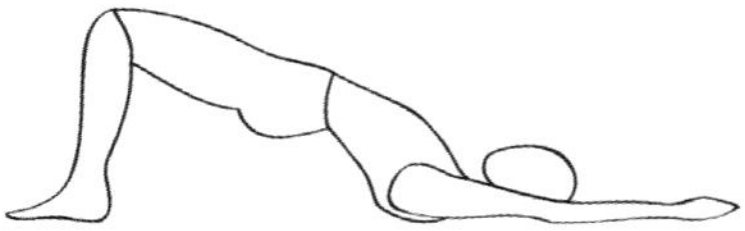

Figure 7.9
Setu Bandha Sarvangasana (Bridge Pose) with block under sacrum

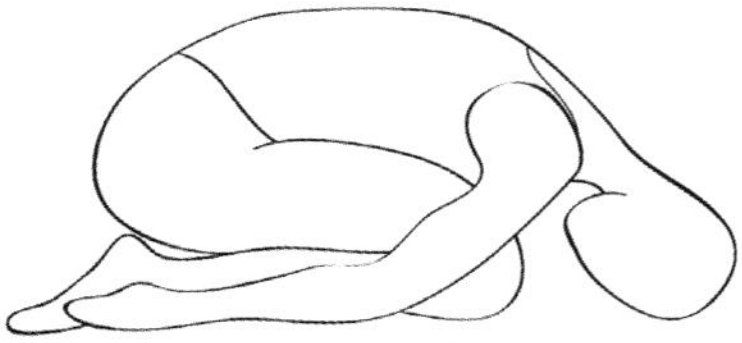

Figure 7.10
Balasana (Child's Pose)

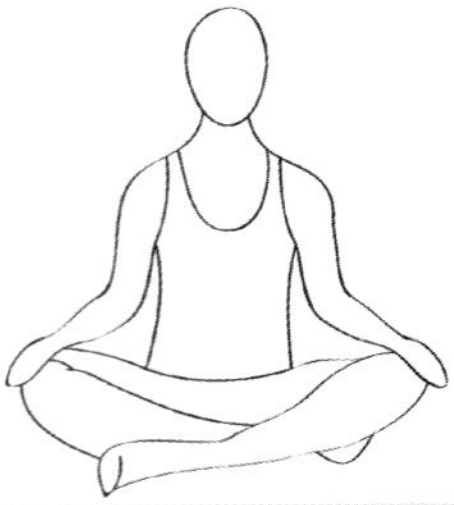

Figure 7.11
Sa Ta Na Ma mantra (in place of relaxation pose)

Yoga Therapy for Sensory Integration Issues 8

"Zach," a 10-year-old boy who has been diagnosed with Autism Spectrum Disorder, social anxiety and selective mutism, is a composite sketch of many children with whom I have worked over the years. Though his pattern of behavior is one of the extremes I have observed in children with Autistic Spectrum Disorder (ASD), his case illustrates how sensory processing issues may show up in the therapy room, and provides a case study of how to interact with a child who may appear disinterested.

Before yoga group, staff forewarned me that Zach, a new boy to the program, did not seem engaged in activities on the unit. He'd been admitted two days previous to an inpatient unit for children with ASD and other pervasive developmental disorders. During his intake assessment, Zach's mother reported that he had an increasingly difficult time going out into the community, and had recently started to hit her when she tried to get him ready. Though Zach's receptive communication skills tested within normal range, he only spoke to family and a very small circle of friends, and only in familiar settings. His social anxiety seemed to be the main trigger for his mutism. As part of his admission, he went through a battery of tests to determine his needs. Some of the tests suggested he processed information very slowly.

As predicted Zach did not participate in yoga and even refused to sit on a yoga mat. Instead he sat in a corner with staff, silently fidgeting with a toy. He attended yoga group again the next week, and again did not participate. But he did sit on a yoga mat with the same toy and played with it silently. By the third week Zach participated in three of the ten yoga poses. He seemed proud of himself as evidenced by the slight smile on his face after he did his first yoga pose. After a month in program, Zach was not only doing most of the yoga poses, but was also helping lead poses (albeit nonverbally). "Leading" for Zach meant pointing to the yoga flash card he wanted to lead, and then placing it in front of his yoga mat as he followed the four steps on the card.

Zach's behavior is indicative of a child whose brain may process information very slowly (Rimland, 1964; Minshew & Goldstein, 1998). Since we will delve deeper into the theories of brain functioning later in the chapter, suffice it to say that researchers like Rimland (1964) and Rogers and Ozonoff (2005) speculate that several symptoms of ASD may be due to *hypo-arousal* of certain parts of the brain. Thus Zach's seeming inattention may not have been due to disinterest, but slow cognitive processing. Perhaps he needed time to familiarize himself with his surroundings, the yoga routine and the expected cues before he could participate. Zach's case is illustrative of the patient observation that a yoga therapist needs to cultivate in order to allow a child with sensory issues to absorb information at his own rate so that he can participate to the best of his ability.

This chapter will explore how pediatric yoga therapy may benefit children with sensory integration issues, cognitive processing issues like Zach's, or attention issues. Children with these symptoms are often diagnosed with ASD, Attention Deficit Hyperactivity Disorder (ADHD), mental retardation (MR), and/or pervasive developmental disorder (PDD), a somewhat dated term now. (As of the DSM-V, the term PDD has been absorbed into the diagnosis of ASD.) For the yoga therapist working with a child who has some of these symptoms or diagnoses, it is important to pay attention to the individual's symptoms and work with those in yoga therapy, *and* to have a general understanding of the diagnoses associated with the symptoms observed.

Yoga therapy is a wonderful adjunctive therapy for sensory integration and attention issues because of its inherently integrative techniques. Galantino, Galbavy and Quinn (2008) reviewed the literature on the therapeutic effects of yoga for children using the *Guide to Physical Therapist Practice* (American Physical Therapy Association, 2003) to gauge the "effectiveness of yoga with respect to practice patterns" (p. 66). Using these standards, Galantino and colleagues (2008) found that yoga may improve "mental ability," (p. 78), motor and social functioning in children with mental challenges. They hypothesized that the reason for this is that "yoga seems to be a multitasking modality that simultaneously treats physical impairments and psychological issues such as stress, anxiety or hyperactivity" (p. 78). For instance, yoga helps one to synchronize movements with the breath, and to build a foundation of simple movements that lead to more subtle and complex poses and movements over time.

Autism Spectrum Disorder

Autism Spectrum Disorder (ASD) is a behaviorally defined neurodevelopmental disorder, meaning it is a collection of symptoms and behaviors reflective of how the brain is processing information (Mandy, Charman & Skuse, 2012). The two main categories of behavioral symptoms in ASD are social communication and restrictive, repetitive behaviors (Mandy, Charman & Skuse, 2012). The Centers for Disease Control (CDC) in the US estimates that one in 68 children is diagnosed with ASD (CDC, 2014), which is an increase from the CDC's estimate just three years previous of one in 88 children (CDC, 2011). The World Health Organization (WHO) estimates the international prevalence as one in 160 children (WHO, 2014). To fit diagnostic criteria, a child must exhibit a certain number of these symptoms and behaviors by a certain age over a period of time. But not all children diagnosed with ASD show the same set of symptoms. For instance, not all individuals who have ASD have cognitive limitations (Child Mind Institute, 2014; WHO, 2014). As such, it is important for a yoga therapist working with children diagnosed with ASD or sensory issues to be aware of individual differences.

Many children diagnosed with ASD, and other neurobehavioral disorders, have issues with *sensory integration* (Rogers & Ozonoff, 2005; National Institute of Neurological Disorders and Stroke, 2014). In her book *Yoga Therapy for Children with Autism and Special Needs* (2013), Louise Goldberg defines sensory integration as "the ability of the brain to receive, organize, and use sensory input in order to participate effectively and satisfactorily in the world" (p. 24). Zach demonstrated this struggle with integrating new sensory in the above vignette. His struggle to organize his sensory input may have slowed his ability to effectively participate in yoga poses for several weeks.

Hypo- and hyper-arousal

In their 2005 paper on the topic, Rogers and Ozonoff refer to sensory integration issues as *sensory dysfunction* (p. 1255). By reviewing the literature, they found that there were two theories as to why an individual experiences sensory dysfunction: either the individual is over-stimulated (hyper-aroused) or under-stimulated (hypo-aroused) by his environment. The theory of *hyper-arousal* (also called "over-arousal") says that 1) a child is more aroused and therefore more reactive to stimuli than normal, and 2) the child is slower to get used to stimuli (e.g., *habituate*). The other theory is of *hypo-arousal* (also called "under-arousal"), which states that a child does not make connections between previous experiences and a current experience, and therefore is not able to generalize his experience. Rogers and Ozonoff (2005) found more evidence for the theory of hypo-arousal as the cause for sensory dysfunction in children with ASD. Using the theory of hypo-arousal, we might conceptualize that Zach took several weeks to participate in yoga, because his nervous system was not stimulated *enough* by the new environment. Thus, it took several weeks of repeated exposure to make the neural connections that allowed him to actively participate.

Attention Deficit Hyperactivity Disorder

Like ASD, ADHD is classified as a neurodevelopmental disorder (Rabiner, 2014). The two broad behavioral criteria for ADHD are inattention and hyperactivity. Goldberg (2013) points out that many children with special needs, including ASD, have symptoms of or are diagnosed with ADHD. Children with attention deficits and ADHD fidget a lot and become distracted easily. They have a hard time waiting their turn, listening and following directions, and curbing impulses to talk or move.

The diagnosis of and medicating of ADHD have become a controversial issue in regions around the world (Partridge, Lucke & Hall, 2014), but especially in the US (Koerth-Baker, 2013; Schwarz & Cohen, 2013; Rabiner, 2014). Several *New York Times* articles have cited a large increase in the number of ADHD diagnoses. *New York Times* writer Maggie Koerth-Baker (2013) found that the incidence of ADHD diagnoses increased from about 5% in the 1990s to its current level of 11%. On the Attention Deficit Disorder Association's website, Dr. David Rabiner (2014) notes that many in the field are concerned that ADHD "is simply a medical term inappropriately attached to children who show largely 'typical' behavior" (Attention Deficit Disorder website, 2014). However, brain studies have shown that those diagnosed with ADHD are different from those who are not (Koerth-Baker, 2013).

Nonetheless, the concern about an increase in the number of ADHD diagnoses has been made greater by the DSM-V's updated definition of ADHD, which has lowered the threshold of symptom severity required for an individual to receive the diagnosis. As a result of this change in the DSM-V definition, *New York Times* writers Alan Schwarz and Sarah Cohen report that ". . . more teenagers are likely to be prescribed medication in the near future" (Cohen & Schwarz, 2013). Speculation about the cause of this increase runs the gamut from US education policies that put an emphasis on standardized test scores (Koerth-Baker, 2013) to food additives (Mayo Clinic, 2014). Public perception that children diagnosed with ADHD are overmedicated is an international concern (Partridge, Lucke & Hall, 2012).

Early Intervention

One popular strategy for addressing both ASD and ADHD treatment is *early intervention.* Early intervention is a term used to describe behavioral strategies used to ameliorate signs and symptoms of a disorder (or disease) early in a child's life (The American Heritage Medical Dictionary, 2007). Early intervention strategies may lessen behavioral symptoms that could later be diagnosed as ASD (Rogers & Vismara, 2008) or ADHD (ADD Treatment Centers, 2005), and therefore are important when addressing these diagnoses and their symptomology. The ADD Treatment Centers website (2005) featured an article entitled *Can ADHD be Prevented in Early Intervention?* "(T)he authors . . . wondered whether early intervention by non-pharmacologic methods might be effective in reducing the number of children showing these early signs who go on to develop ADHD" (online, 2005). The National Institute of Neurological Disorders and Stroke (2014) says that early intervention is key to helping children with sensory and attention issues to optimize their potential.

Yoga therapy offers a holistic, non-pharmaceutical option that can complement other early intervention strategies for children and adolescents showing signs of ASD, ADHD, MR and/or PDD to maximize their skills.

Yoga for sensory integration, cognitive processing and attention issues

Yoga treatments for children and adolescents with sensory integration, cognitive processing and attention issues have a lot in common. Children with these issues benefit from consistent routines, clear and simple instructions that are repeated, breaking skills down into small steps, learning how to sequence tasks appropriately, and being rewarded when the task is complete (Goldberg, 2013). Louise Goldberg is the founder of Creative Relaxation ®, a pediatric yoga therapy designed specifically for children with ASD and other special needs. We will explore the key elements to creating a therapeutic yoga session for this population by applying some of Goldberg's recommendations, as well as an evidenced-based method used at Children's Hospital Colorado.

Children with ASD, and many with ADHD, benefit from visual schedules (Bryan & Gast, 2000) when learning new tasks. The Neuropsychiatric Special Care Unit (NSCU) at Children's Hospital Colorado provides services to children with ASD and other neurodevelopmental issues. The NSCU structures the hospital environment using the TEACCH (Treatment and Education of Autistic and related Communication Handicapped Children) model in its treatment approach (Gabriels et al., 2012; Siegel & Gabriels, 2014). Developed at the University of North Carolina (UNC) Chapel Hill by Eric Schopler and colleagues, the TEACCH model uses visual schedules to help individuals with ASD learn and practice sequences of tasks.

Gabriels and colleagues (2012) say, "the environmental organization is necessary to decrease the need for excessive physical prompting" (p. 3). A yoga therapist can easily incorporate visual structure in the yoga environment following a few simple steps: Arrange the mats and create a visual schedule of the yoga practice before the yoga session begins. Using flashcards of yoga poses is an excellent way to create a visual schedule. Several yoga flashcard sets for children are available online and in bookstores. My personal favorite is *Yoga Pretzels*® (Guber & Kalish, 2005), because the illustrations are simple and colorful, and every pose has four instructions (this helps with consistency and simplicity). If I don't have a card for a particular activity, I use an object to represent it. For instance, I will place a tennis ball between two cards to signify that we will massage the bottom of our feet with a tennis ball at that point in the practice.

I reinforce the visual cues with simple verbal instruction. For example, as Zach and his peers walked into the yoga room and saw the yoga mats in a line, I said, "Ok, guys, first take a seat on a yoga mat." TEACCH uses a verbal instruction method referred to as "First, then" verbal sequencing (Beaudette & Harhen, 2008). Thus, once I saw the boys were sitting on their yoga mats I said, "**First**, let's look at the yoga cards laid out in front of you. **Then** we'll practice them together." Creating these elements of visual and verbal organization and structure in the yoga environment cultivates an atmosphere of safety and predictability for the group.

Goldberg (2013) says it is important to make yoga therapy fun for children with special needs. In my experience, many children with ASD and ADHD enjoy leading the rest of their peers in poses. It seems to make them feel more involved and it also teaches them how to follow, which can be a challenging task for children with ASD. The *Yoga Pretzels*® flashcards consistently illustrate four steps for practicing any yoga pose. This consistency makes it easy for children with special needs to lead a yoga pose, even if it is their first time doing yoga. Thus, this is a regular part of my clinical practice with this population.

More than other groups of children, this population will often surprise with skills they develop, or seem to forget. Goldberg (2013) recommends planning for sessions but allowing for changes when the group presents with different needs than the planned session provides. In my clinical practice, I talk with staff before the group starts to find out how participants are getting along and what special needs individuals have. Once I have a sense of the milieu's affect, I decide on a specific yoga intervention. However, if I've decided to lead a very structured group and then find the group is following all directions and shows good teamwork, I will suggest that participants take turns leading. On the other hand, if I find that the group atmosphere chaotic, then I will ring a bell and tell the group that we are going to do a more structured activity led by me.

In her book, Goldberg (2013) refers to 10 Golden Rules of yoga therapy for children with special needs. The final Golden Rule "Keep It Positive" (p. 35) refers to positive reinforcement, a powerful tool in working with children who have special needs. For instance, by paying attention to Zach's behavior each week, I was able to observe positive efforts he continually made. First, he sat quietly throughout the entire first session. Then he joined the group by sitting on a yoga mat. Finally, in the third week, he began to execute the yoga poses. He received encouragement every step of the way from me, the other staff and his peers. This culture of positivity allows for individual strengths and needs to be expressed and celebrated.

In summary

The prevalence of children diagnosed with ASD and ADHD is increasing worldwide, but especially in the US. Regardless of the controversy surrounding these apparent increases, there is a great need to address the symptoms that lead to these two diagnoses. Many in the field advocate for early intervention strategies that are holistic, integrative and non-pharmacologic approaches to treating symptoms. Yoga therapy offers a great adjunctive, early intervention strategy for this population.

A yoga therapist is well equipped to offer a safe, fun, and child-centered yoga practice for children with special needs when armed with training, multi-disciplinary support and experience. In conjunction with the TEACCH model that focuses on consistent routines, visual learning and simplified instructions, Goldberg's yoga method offers children with ASD and ADHD the potential of optimizing their skills and strengths. Refer to Chapter 9 for detailed instructions, modifications and contraindications of the poses.

Practices

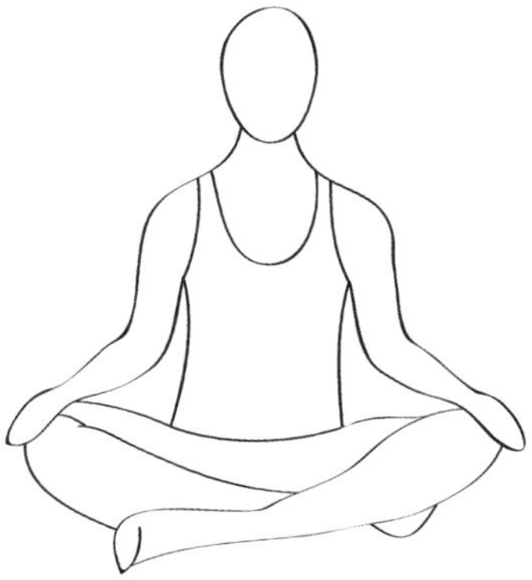

Figure 8.1
Sukhasana (Simple Sitting Pose) with Snake Breath

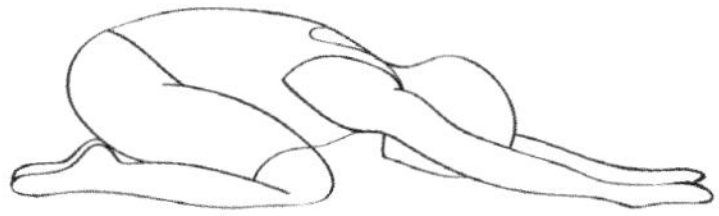

Figure 8.2
Balasana (Child's Pose)

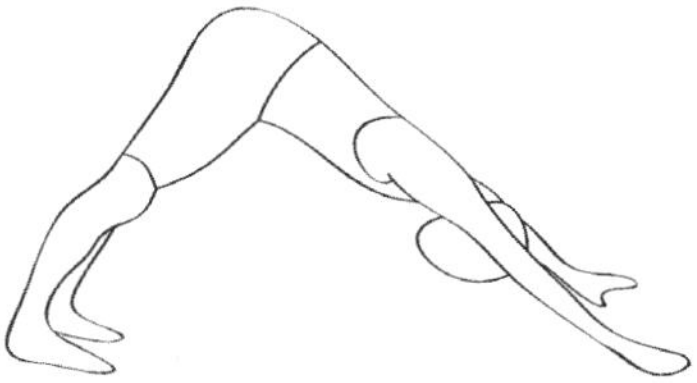

Figure 8.3
Adho Mukha Svanasana (Downward-facing Dog)

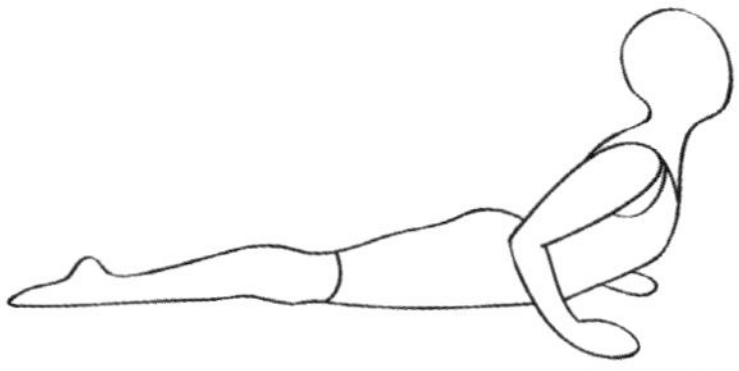

Figure 8.4
Bhujangasana (Cobra Pose)

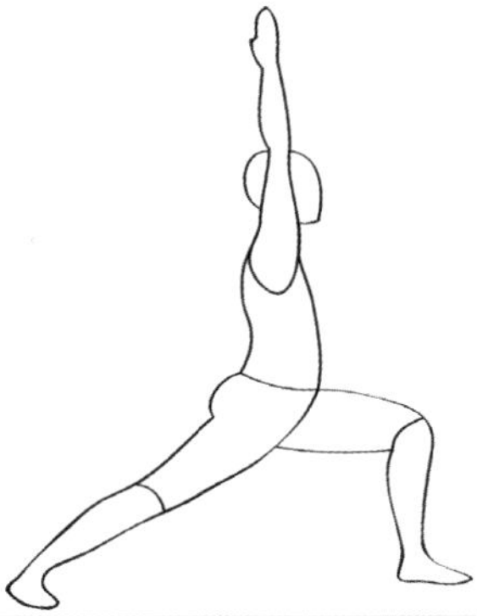

Figure 8.5
Virabhadrasana I (Warrior I)—repeat on both sides

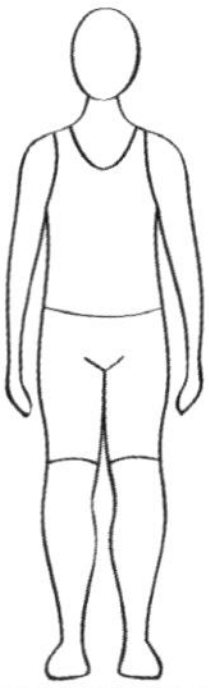

Figure 8.6
Tadasana (Mountain Pose)

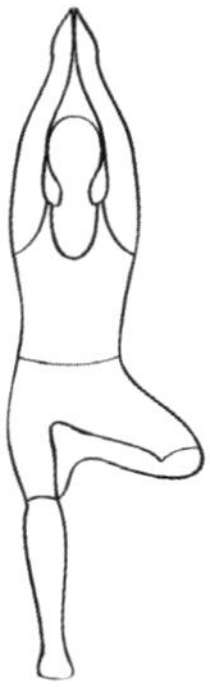

Figure 8.7
Vrksasana (Tree Pose)—repeat on both sides

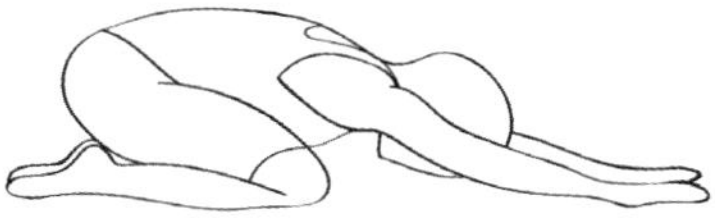

Figure 8.8
Balasana (Child's Pose)

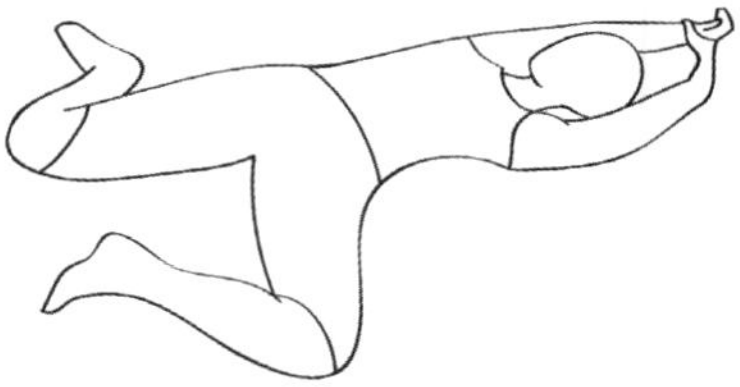

Figure 8.9
Windshield wipers

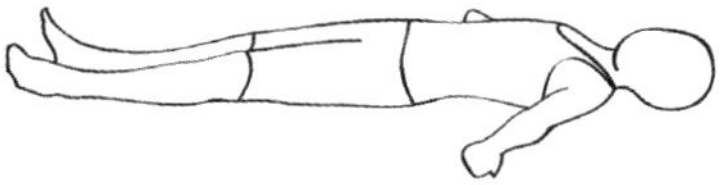

Figure 8.10
Savasana with beanie baby, or other soft, weighted object on belly to feel breathing

Practice Library

9

Poses are listed alphabetically with their Sanskrit name first, followed by the common translation and then a kid-friendly name that can be used with school-aged children. Just the kid-friendly name is listed when it is the same as the common name. It is best to use the common translation or Sanskrit name with adolescents to respect developmental maturity. There are a few poses that do not have traditional Sanskrit names (e.g. Windshield Wipers Pose). In this case the common English name is given.

Most poses feature modifications for the classic form of the pose. The particular modifications listed in this book are common adjustments either needed for growing bodies or in the case of injury. In other cases where modifications are given, it is simply a matter of personal preference, as is the case with Balasana. Additionally, some poses are dynamic and have more than one movement, such as Apanasana. In this case, two illustrations depict the main movements. Dynamic movements coordinated with the breath are traditionally called a vinyasa, or sequence of poses linked by breath (Ezraty, 2007). Thus, the term vinyasa throughout this practice library refers to this coordination of movement with breath from one position to another.

Brief descriptions of breathing practices used throughout the sample practices are listed before pose illustrations. Also, brief descriptions of the relaxation and visualizations used throughout the text are listed after the illustrations.

Breathing techniques

Balloon Breath (for pre-schoolers and school-aged children)

- Inhale, imagine filling up a colored balloon with air and see your body filling up with the same color
- Exhale, and imagine the balloon slowly losing air, feel your body relax and let go
- Repeat 10 times

Birthday Candle Breath (for pre-schoolers and school-aged children)

- Spread the fingers of one or both hands out in front of you like birthday candles
- Inhale deeply
- Exhale by blowing on your fingers, as if you're blowing out the candles on a birthday cake!
- Repeat 5 times

Box Breathing (for school-aged children)

- Hold index finger in the air, as if it's a colored pencil
- Inhale, and "draw" a line across to the right
- Exhale, draw a line down
- Inhale draw a line across to the left
- Exhale, draw a line up to complete the box
- Repeat 5 times

Counting Breath (for school-aged children and adolescents)

- Notice the breath coming in and going out
- Inhale, notice the expansive, opening, lengthening qualities of the inhale
- Exhale, notice the dropping, rooting, grounding qualities of the exhale
- Notice that the breath naturally slows down as you bring awareness to it

- Count how long your next inhalation is
- Exhale, to the same count
- Every time the mind wanders, just bring it back to the simple count of the breath
- School-aged children can do this practice for up to a minute; adolescents can do it for up to 5 minutes

Ocean Breath (for school-aged children and adolescents)

- Feel the wavelike quality of the breath
- Inhale, feel the breath rise and fill the belly and chest like the crest of a wave
- Exhale, feel the breath drop like the trough of a wave
- School-aged children can do this practice for up to a minute; adolescents can do it for up to 5 minutes

Snake Breath (older pre-schoolers and school-aged children)

- What does a snake sound like?
- Everyone hiss like a snake!
- Make the hiss as long as possible
- Repeat 5 times

Viloma Breathing (best for adolescents)

For depression: split the exhale into three parts.

For anxiety: split the inhale into three parts.

- Notice the breath coming in and going out
- Inhale, imagine the torso is like a cup filling up with water from the bottom to the top
- Exhale, imagine the breath is like water pouring out of the cup from the top to the bottom
- Inhale a third of the way, filling the bottom of the belly and hold breath; inhale another third, filling the mid-ribs and hold breath; inhale the last third filling the upper chest
- Exhale, let all the air out slowly and completely
- Repeat for 1–3 minutes

Yoga poses

Adho Mukha Svanasana
Kid-friendly name: Downward-facing Dog

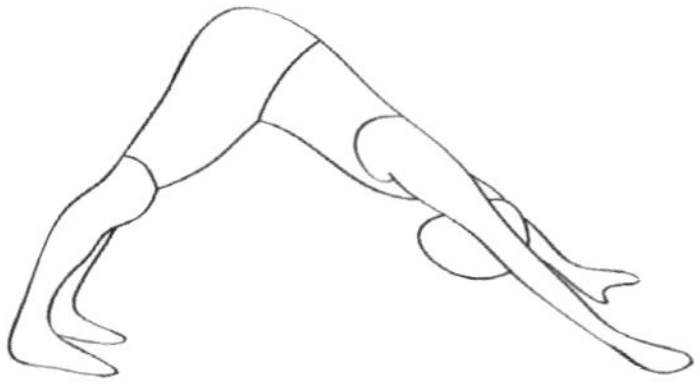

1. Come onto all fours, shrug shoulders up and back.
2. **Inhale,** lift hips.
3. **Exhale,** and extend legs back (most people, kids and adults, do not get heels to the floor); three things to watch for: a hunched back, "scrunched" shoulders and hyperextension in the knees.
4. **Inhale,** roll shoulders back, lift hips up and back.
5. **Exhale,** spin inner thighs towards back wall to lengthen the back.

School-aged children: stay 5–10 breaths

Adolescents: can stay up to 60 seconds, depending on strength

Where do you feel it? Calves, hamstrings, shoulders, anywhere along the spine (depends on individual's flexibility)

Benefits: Lengthens back; stretches legs; tones belly; energizes body and mind; adolescents may feel the subtle "scooping" in and up of the lower belly during the exhale in this pose (which is the beginnings of a subtle yoga hold known as *udhyana bandha*)

Contraindications: wrist weakness/repetitive strain (such as carpal tunnel); diarrhea; high blood pressure or headache; dizziness or nausea

***Adho Mukha Svanasana* modifications**

- This is a tough pose; some teachers say it's three poses in one—a forward bend, a standing pose and an arm balance

- Most people (children, adolescents and adults) need to bend knees, allowing heels to lift in order to get desired stretch in back and neck

Apanasana Vinyasa
Knees to Chest Pose
Kid-friendly name: Knees to Chest Pose

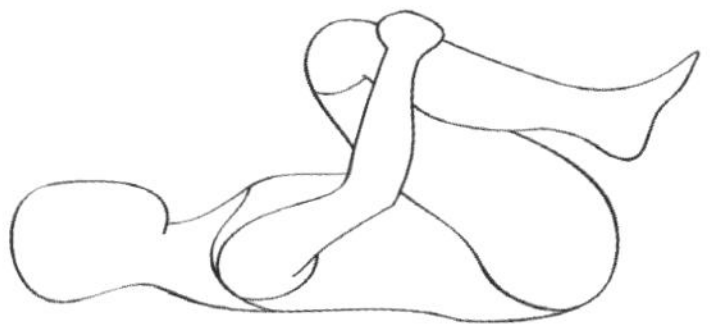

1 While lying on back, **exhale** while drawing bent knees to chest.

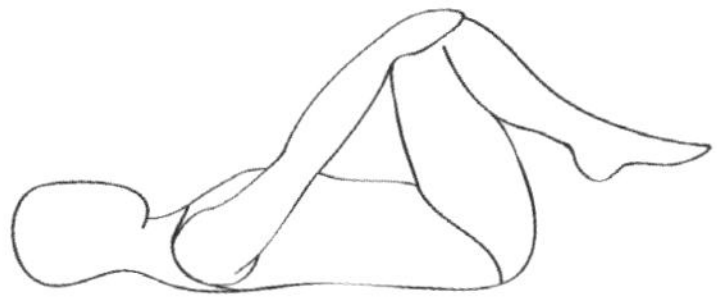

2 **Inhale,** while pressing knees away from body to straighten arms.
3 Repeat the vinyasa from A to B 5–10 times.

School-aged children repeat up to 5 times. Adolescents repeat up to 10 times.

Where do you feel it? Low back; hips
Benefits: Massages lower back and stomach, relieves gas, releases hip tension, circulates blood through lower back
Contraindications: knee issues; soft tissue sensitivity on back; diarrhea

***Apanasana* modifications**
- For knee issues: Place hands on thighs behind knees
- For soft tissue sensitivity in back or hips: Lie on blankets

Baddha Konasana A
Bound Angle Pose A
Kid-friendly name: Cobbler's Pose A

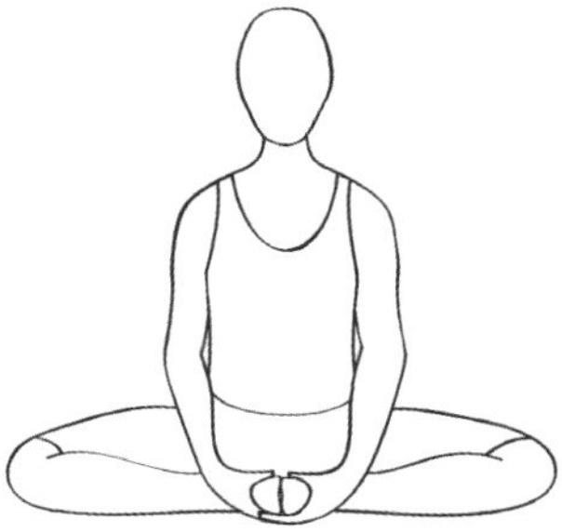

1 Sit up tall.
2 Bring soles of feet together (feet as far away from body as allows shoulders to stay directly above hips).
3 **Inhale,** roll shoulders up and back.
4 **Exhale,** take hold of feet with hands (if possible).

School-aged children and adolescents can stay in the pose for 5–10 breaths, as long as no tightness is felt in the joints (sometimes adolescents are tighter due to growing pains and sports that tighten their muscles. Encourage them to listen to their bodies to determine their capacity, and perhaps only stay for 5 breaths.)

Where do you feel it? Hips, back
Benefits: Lengthens hamstrings; stretches back
Contraindications: Hip, knee or back injury/strain

***Baddha Konasana* modifications**
- For tight hamstrings or back: Move feet away from body until shoulder can track over hips
- For very flexible individuals: Allow inner feet to come apart, keeping outside edges together, like an open book

Baddha Konasana B
Bound Angle Pose B
Kid-friendly name: Cobbler's Pose B

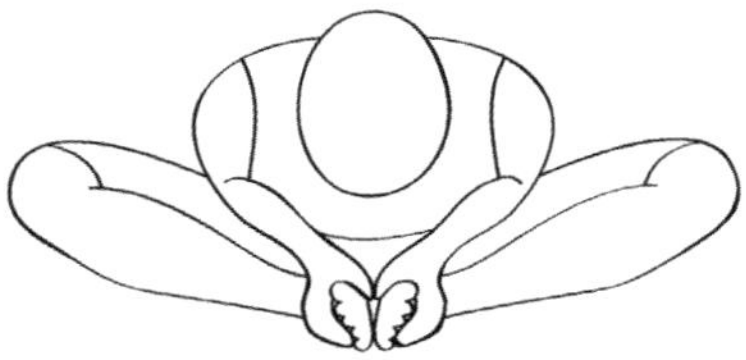

1. Sit in *Baddha Konasana A.*
2. **Exhale,** leaning forward as much as hips and knees will allow.
3. **Inhale,** roll shoulders up towards ceiling and back away from ears.
4. **Exhale,** let head fall forward as far as is comfortable for neck and shoulders.

School-aged children and adolescents can both stay in the pose for 5–10 breaths, as long as no tightness is felt in the joints (sometimes adolescents are tighter due to growing pains and sports that tighten their muscles. Encourage them to listen to their bodies to determine their capacity, and perhaps only stay 5 breaths.)

Where do you feel it? Hips, back, legs
Benefits: Stretches hips and back
Contraindications: Hip, knee or back injury/strain; pregnant

***Baddha Konasana* modifications**

- For tight hamstrings or back: Only lean forward as far as feels intense but comfortable (e.g. no pain)

Balasana
Child's Pose
Kid-friendly name: Rock Pose

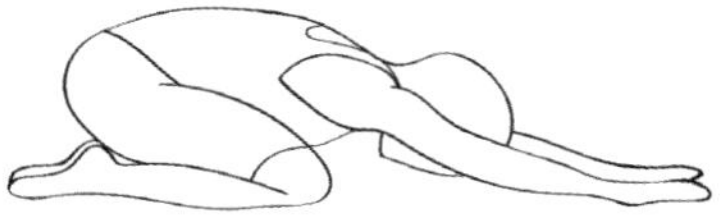

1. **Inhale** while sitting on knees, big toes together and knees apart.
2. **Exhale** and slide hands out in front on body, rest belly on legs.

Allow school-aged children to stay in the pose for less than 10 breaths. Keep adolescents in the pose for 10+ breaths.

Where do you feel it? Back, hips, ankles
Benefits: Gently stretches the hips, thighs and ankles; lengthens spine, which can relieve pain or tension in neck and back when head and torso are supported; calming, stress-relieving pose
Contraindications: Knee issues/injuries; diarrhea; pregnancy

***Balasana* modifications**
Benefits: Good when neck, shoulder or hip tightness prevents relaxation in other positions

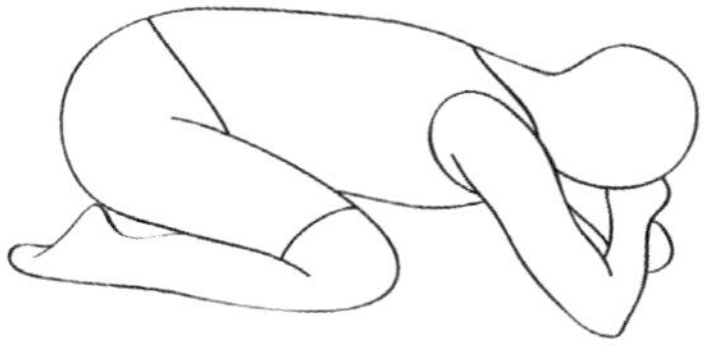

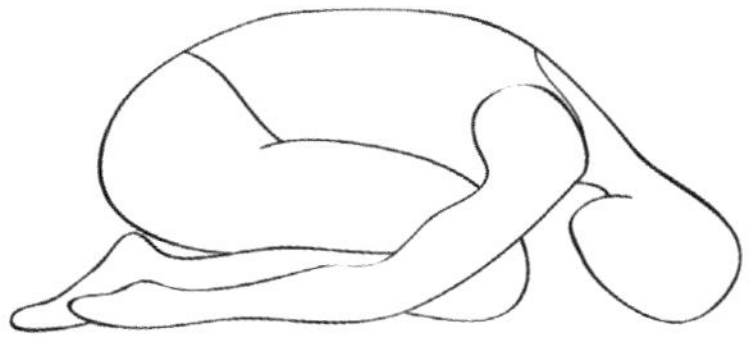

Benefits: Relieves tension in trapezius muscles of shoulders

Bhujangasana
Kid-friendly name: Cobra Pose

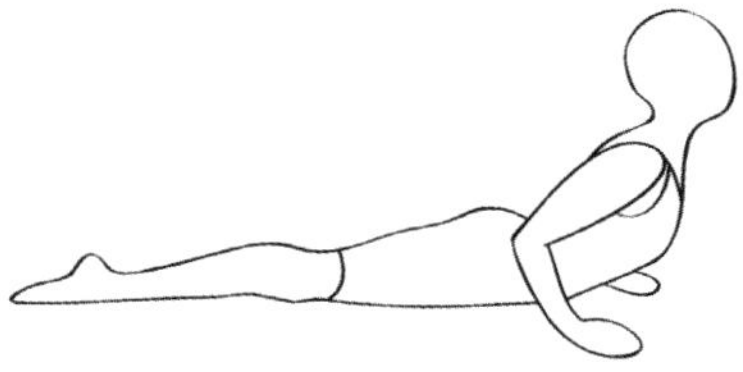

1. Lie on belly with hands pressing floor beneath shoulders.
2. **Inhale** and raise head, chest and shoulders.
3. **Exhale** and extend tailbone towards heels.
4. **Inhale** rolling shoulders up and back.
5. **Exhale** to come out of pose.

Kid-friendly modification: Hiss when coming out of pose.
School-aged children stay in the pose for 3–5 breaths. Adolescents stay for 5–10 breaths.

Where do you feel it? Lower back, shoulders, increase in energy level
Benefits: Energizing pose; strengthens spinal muscles; stretches chest, lungs, shoulders, and abdomen; firms the buttocks; stimulates abdominal organs; expands the heart and lungs; relieves sciatica
Contraindications: Lower back, shoulder or neck pain/injuries; pregnancy

***Bhujangasana* modification**
Sphinx Pose

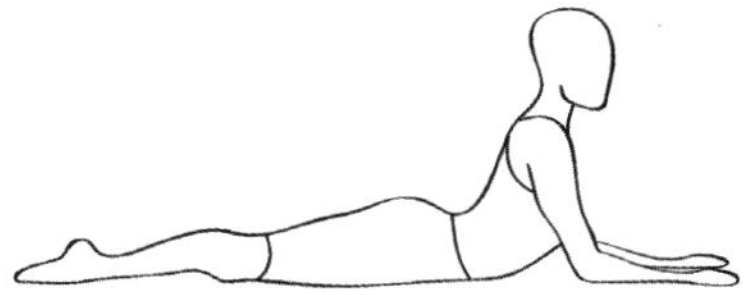

Benefits: Back stretch for those with lower back pain

Dikasana B (or Virabhadrasana III)
Warrior III
Kid-friendly name: Airplane Pose

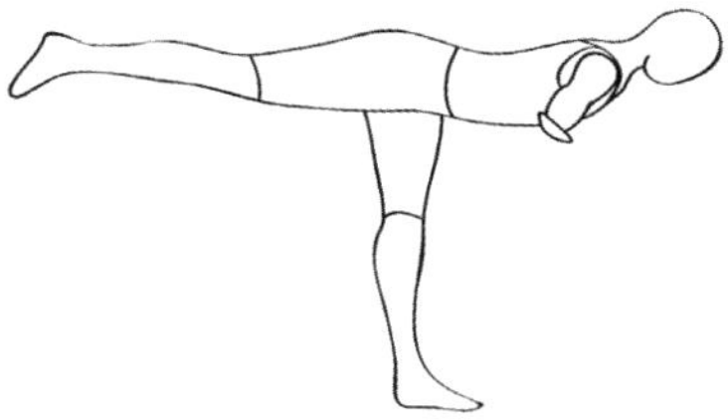

1. Stand in *Tadasana.*
2. **Exhale** and extend right leg back reaching big toe to the floor.
3. **Inhale** and extend arms up to the sky.
4. **Exhale** and lean forward until right big toe hovers above floor.
5. **Inhale** and extend arms out to the side (as in the figure above).
6. Repeat on other side for equal number of breaths or counts.

School-aged children stay in the pose for 3–5 breaths. Adolescents stay for 5–10 breaths.

Where do you feel it? Supporting leg, back, core, shoulders, arms, confidence

Benefits: Increases confidence and concentration; cultivates balance; strengthens ankles and legs; tones belly, shoulders and back
Contraindications: High blood pressure; major hip, knee or ankle injuries that continue to cause pain/distress

***Dikasana* modifications**

- For balance issues: Keep back toes on the floor
- For greater challenge: Extend arms out in front (classic Virabhadrasana III form)

Eka Pada Rajakapotasana
Prep One-Footed Royal Pigeon Pose Prep
Kid-friendly name: Pigeon Pose

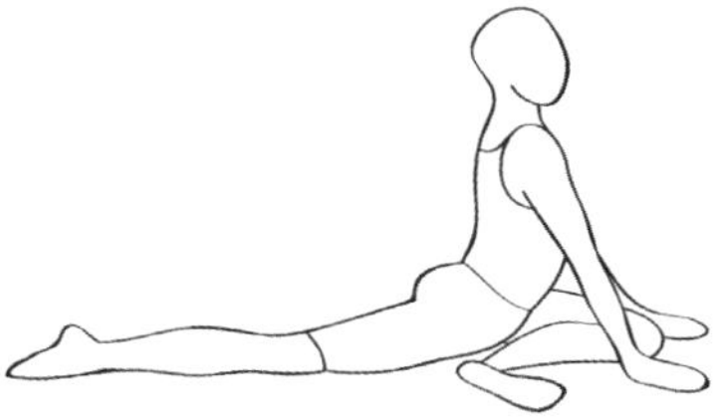

1 Come onto all fours.
2 **Exhale,** cross right shin in front of left knee.
3 **Inhale,** lift chest and roll shoulders back.
4 **Exhale,** extend left leg back as in the illustration above.
5 Keep hips level (i.e. don't let right hip sink onto floor lower than left hip).
6 Repeat on other side for equal number of breaths or counts.

School-aged children and adolescents can both stay in each side of the pose for up to 30 seconds, as long as no tightness is felt in the joints (sometimes adolescents are tighter due to growing pains and sports that tighten their muscles. Encourage them to listen to their bodies to determine their capacity, and perhaps only stay 5 breaths on each side.)

Where do you feel it? Bent-knee hip, lower back stretch
Benefits: Increases hip flexibility and mobility; loosens back
Contraindications: Knee, ankle or sacroiliac injuries (or extreme tightness in one or more of these areas)

***Eka Pada Rajakapotasana* modifications**

- For tight hips and knee issues: Place block beneath bent-knee hip

Garudasana
Kid-friendly name: Eagle Pose

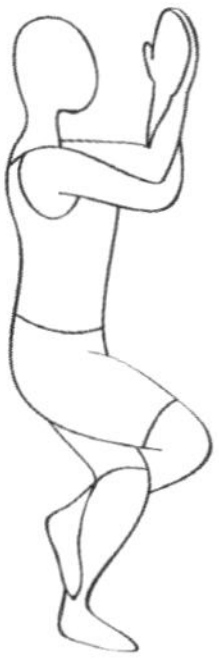

1 Stand in *Tadasana*, Mountain Pose.
2 **Exhale,** slightly bend knees and cross left leg over right.
3 **Inhale,** extend arms and cross right arm over left.
4 **Exhale,** bend both elbows and "catch" bottom of right hand with left fingers/hand, while bending knees more (if possible).
5 Repeat on other side for equal number of breaths or counts.

School-aged children stay in the pose for 3–10 breaths, depending on balance and coordination. Adolescents stay for 10 or more breaths, also depending on balance and coordination.

Where do you feel it? Release in hips, knees, shoulders; increased vigor
Benefits: Increases confidence and concentration; cultivates balance; strengthens ankles and legs; tones belly, shoulders and back; releases tension while coming out of pose
Contraindications: Knee, ankle or hip injuries

***Garudasana* modifications**

- For balance issues: Place foot (that would be wrapped around standing leg) on floor

Gomukhasana Arms
Ear-of-the-Cow Arms
Kid Friendly Name: Chicken Wing

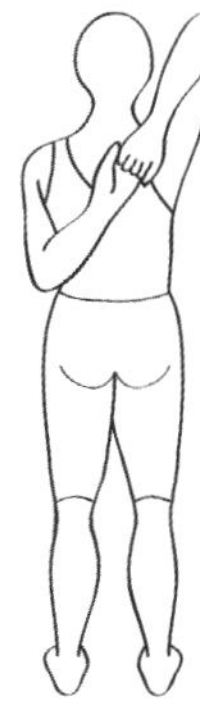

1. Stand in *Tadasana*, Mountain Pose.
2. **Exhale,** roll shoulders up and back.
3. **Inhale,** extend right arm to sky.
4. **Exhale,** bend right elbow and grab right hand with left hand behind the back.
5. Repeat on other side for equal number of breaths or counts.

School-aged children stay in the pose for 3–5 breaths. Adolescents stay for 10 breaths, depending on shoulder flexi bility (which can vary greatly from one adolescent to another).

Where do you feel it? Triceps, shoulders, chest
Benefits: Stretches triceps and shoulders
Contraindications: Shoulder, wrist, elbow injury

***Gomukhasana Arm* modification**
Chicken Wing

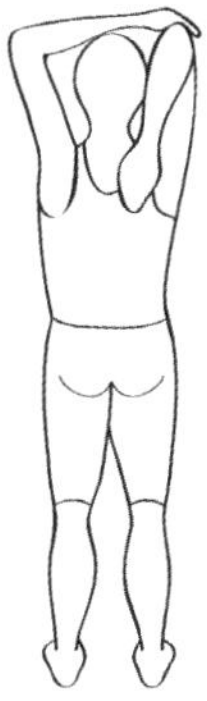

Benefits: Stretches triceps and shoulders, especially if tight

Hamstring Stretch
Kid-friendly name: Runner's Stretch

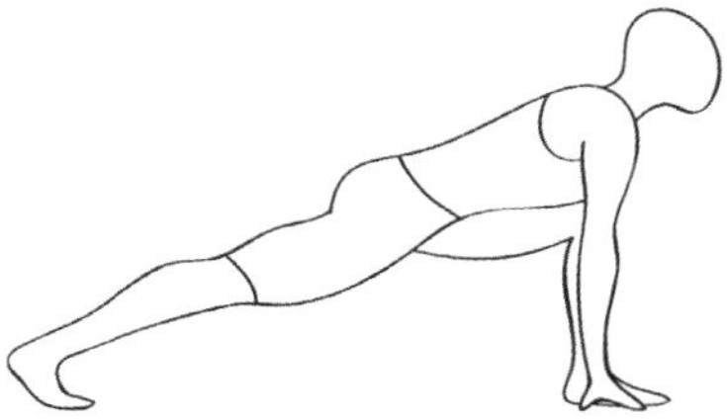

1. Come onto all fours
2. **Exhale,** extend flexed right foot forward and lean back until finger tips press floor (use blocks if fingers don't reach floor).
3. **Inhale,** reach chest forward and up, rolling shoulders back and down.
4. **Exhale,** resist the stretch by pulling extended head towards body as if about to come out of the pose (this protects the knee and hamstring from overstretching).
5. Repeat on other side for equal number of breaths or counts.

School-aged children and adolescents can both stay on each side of the pose for 5–10 breaths, as long as no tightness is felt in the joints (sometimes adolescents are tighter due to growing pains and sports that tighten their muscles. Encourage them to listen to their bodies to determine their capacity, and perhaps only stay 5 breaths on each side).

Where do you feel it? Back of leg, lower back, hips
Benefits: Lengthens hamstrings; stretches hip
Contraindications: Knee or hamstring injuries or strain

Hamstring Stretch modifications

- For tight hamstrings: Bend extended knee more.

Hastasana
Kid-friendly name: Waterfall Pose

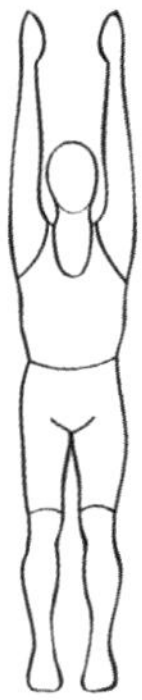

1. Stand in *Tadasana*, Mountain Pose
2. **Exhale,** roll shoulders up and back
3. **Inhale,** extend both arms to sky
4. **Exhale,** press down through legs, feel feet ground into floor

School-aged children stay in the pose for 3–5 breaths. Adolescents stay for 10 breaths, depending on shoulder flexibility (which can vary greatly from one adolescent to another).

Where do you feel it? Shoulders, back
Benefits: Stretches shoulders and back; helps with balance
Contraindications: Shoulder injury

***Hastasana* modifications**

- For tight shoulders (or to teach good shoulder alignment): Bend elbows so that they are in line with shoulder like a football goal pose

Janu Sirsasana A
Head-to-Knee Pose
Kid-friendly name: Runner's Stretch

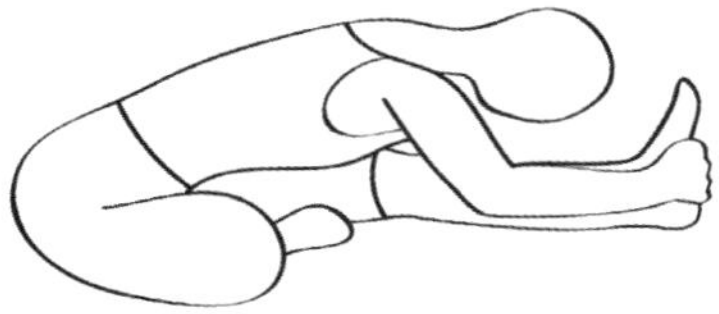

1. Sit with legs extended.
2. **Exhale,** bend right knee placing right foot anywhere along left leg, making sure that both sitting bones are on the ground.
3. **Inhale,** extend arms up to the sky.
4. **Exhale,** reach arms towards left foot (again, making sure both sitting bones are grounded).
5. Repeat on other side for equal number of breaths or counts.

School-aged children and adolescents can both stay for 5–10 breaths on each side of the pose, as long as no tightness is felt in the joints (sometimes adolescents are tighter due to growing pains and sports that tighten their muscles. Encourage them to listen to their bodies to determine their capacity, and perhaps only stay 5 breaths on each side.)

Where do you feel it? Back of leg, lower back, hip
Benefits: Lengthens hamstrings; stretches back
Contraindications: Hamstring or back injuries or strain

Janu Sirsasana modifications

- Bend extended leg if legs are tight

Lunge
Kid-friendly name: Lunge

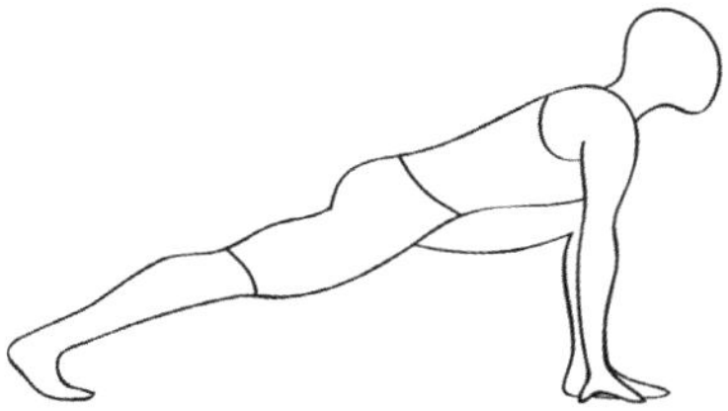

1 Come onto all fours.
2 **Exhale,** extend left leg straight back with foot flexed (toes turned under).
3 **Inhale,** reach chest towards center of the room and roll shoulders back.
4 **Exhale,** reach through back heel.
5 Repeat on other side for equal number of breaths or counts.

School-aged children and adolescents can both stay for 10–20 seconds on each side of the pose depending on strength and flexibility.

Where do you feel it? Hamstrings, hips, back, back of leg
Benefits: Stretches hamstrings and back; strengthens and stretches hips
Contraindications: Ankle or knee injuries

Lunge modifications

- For serious ankle or knee injuries: avoid this pose
- For less stretch in the back leg or knee strain on front leg: bend back knee to floor

Marichyasana C
Pose to Marichi
Kid-friendly name: Seated Twist

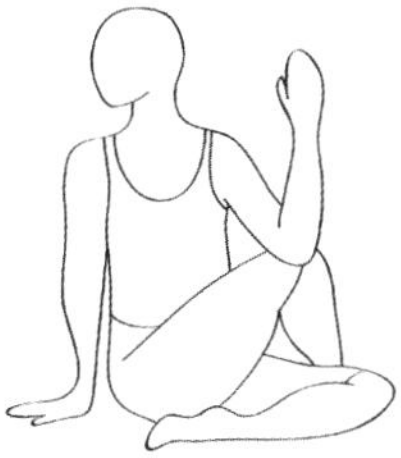

1 Sit with legs extended.
2 **Exhale,** bend right knee, crossing right foot to outside of left leg, and then cross left leg so that left foot touches right buttock.
3 **Inhale,** lift chest and roll shoulders back.
4 **Exhale,** cross left elbow on the outside of right knee.
5 **Inhale,** lengthen through spine.
6 **Exhale,** twist lower belly to back wall.
7 **Inhale,** re-lengthen through spine.
8 **Exhale,** twist mid ribs toward back wall.
9 **Inhale,** re-lengthen through spine.
10 **Exhale,** turn head and neck toward back wall (unless you have a neck injury).
11 Repeat on other side for equal number of breaths or counts.

School-aged children hold the pose for 3–5 breaths on each side. Adolescents can stay on each side of the pose for 5–8 breaths

Where do you feel it? Back, shoulders, hips
Benefits: Stretches hamstrings and back; strengthens and stretches hips
Contraindications: Herniated disc or other spinal injury; ankle injuries; pregnancy

Marichyasana **C modification**

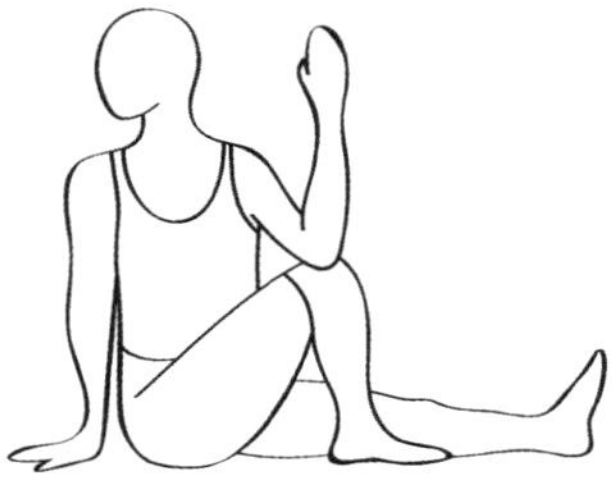

Benefits: Relieves pressure in lower leg; allows spine to lengthen if back is tight

Paripurna Navasana
Kid-friendly name: Boat Pose

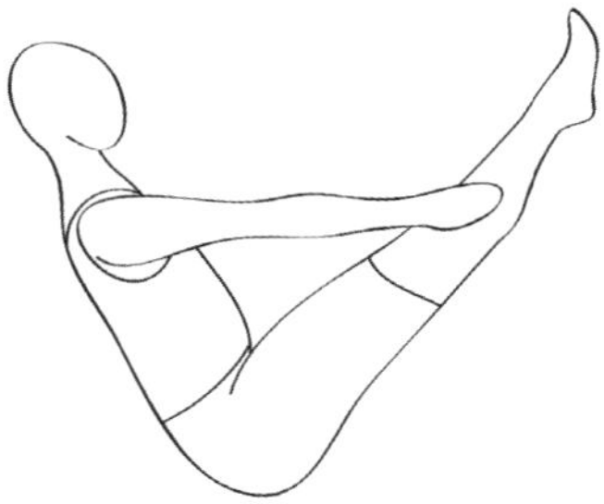

1. Sit with knees bent, feet on floor.
2. With hands holding backs of knees, lean back until toes hover slightly off the floor.
3. **Exhale,** draw lower belly in and lift feet so they're as high as the knees.
4. **Inhale,** extend legs as in picture above.

School-aged children and adolescents demonstrate a wide range of abilities in this pose. If it's difficult for a child or adolescent, start by holding the pose for 5 breaths. For strong school-aged children, sing "Row, Row, Row Your Boat" as a fun way to help them build core strength. Strong adolescents have fun making it a contest of who can stay up longest (up to 1 minute).

Where do you feel it? Core, legs, arms
Benefits: Strengthens core, hip flexors and back; improves digestion; relieves stress (especially when singing in pose!)
Contraindications: Lower back injury or strain; asthma; diarrhea; menstruation; headache; heart problems; low blood pressure; insomnia; pregnancy

Paripurna Navasana **modification**

- Core-strengthening poses can be very beneficial for those with mild lower back strain. Instruct child or adolescent to hold pose at steps 2 or 3, whichever helps engage abdominal muscles without causing strain in lower back.
- For lower back issues: Place hands on floor behind hips

Parivrtta Trikonasana
Revolved Triangle
Kid-friendly name: Revolved Triangle

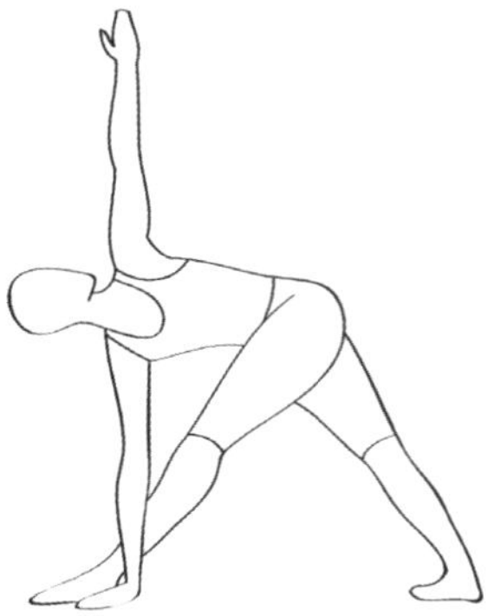

1. Stand in *Tadasana,* Mountain Pose.
2. **Exhale,** place hands on hips and step left leg back with toes angled towards side of mat, heel on floor (hips now face "front" right foot and leg).
3. **Inhale,** roll shoulders back, extend left arm to sky and continue to rotate right hip back so that hips are square to the front of the mat.
4. **Exhale,** reach left hand down to right leg to whatever depth allows the spine to stay lengthened and aligned.

5 Repeat on the other side for equal number of breaths or counts.

School-aged children and adolescents can both stay in each side of the pose for 5–10 breaths, as long as no tightness is felt in the joints (sometimes adolescents are tighter due to growing pains and sports that tighten their muscles. Encourage them to listen to their bodies to determine their capacity, and perhaps only stay 5 breaths on each side.)

Where do you feel it? Outer legs, calves, hips, back
Benefits: Strengthens and stretches legs; stretches hips; relieves mild back pain; opens chest for fuller breathing; strengthens abdominal organs; increases sense of balance
Contraindications: Should be done with the instruction/assistance of an experienced yoga teacher or therapist; also do not practice this pose in cases of back injury or strain; diarrhea; menstruation; headache; low blood pressure; insomnia; pregnancy

***Parivrtta Trikonasana* modification**
- Don't extend top arm—place it on hips to help square hips towards front of mat
- Place hands on either side of front foot (or on blocks or floor)

Parsvottanasana
Intense Side Stretch
Kid-friendly name: Pyramid Pose

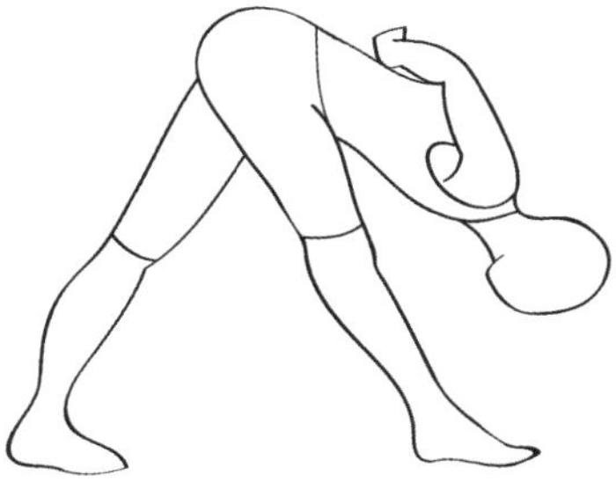

1 Stand in *Tadasana*, Mountain Pose.
2 **Exhale,** place hands on hips and step left leg back with toes angled towards side of mat, heel on floor (hips now face "front" right foot and leg).
3 **Inhale,** roll shoulders back, look up toward the ceiling and clasp elbows behind back.
4 **Exhale,** lengthen torso towards right leg.
5 Repeat on other side for equal number of breaths or counts.

School-aged children and adolescents can both stay in each side of the pose for 5–10 breaths, as long as no tightness is felt in the joints (sometimes adolescents are tighter due to growing pains and sports that tighten their muscles. Encourage them to listen to their bodies to determine their capacity, and perhaps only stay 5 breaths on each side.)

Where do you feel it? Back of leg, hips, spine
Benefits: Strengthens and stretches legs; stretches hips; relieves mild back pain; improves balance
Contraindications: Hamstring injury; pregnancy

***Parsvottanasana* modifications**
- Place hands on either side of front foot (either on blocks or floor)
- For hamstring or gluteal injury: Bend front knee slightly

Paschimottanasana
Kid-friendly name: Seated Forward Fold

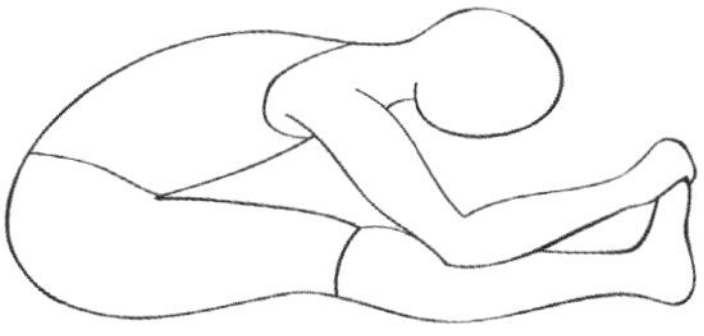

1 Sit with legs extended, flex feet – toes point towards ceiling.
2 **Inhale,** lengthen through the spine.
3 **Exhale,** extend torso over legs, reaching hands for outer shins, ankles or feet (keeping elbows slightly bent).

4 **Inhale,** reach chest up and roll shoulders back.
5 **Exhale,** reach through back heal, slightly digging heals into floor to engage back leg. Muscles.

School-age children can stay in the pose for 5–10 breaths; adolescents can stay 10–60 seconds, depending on flexibility and comfort.

Where do you feel it? Low back and middle of hamstring muscles
Benefits: Stretches hamstrings and back; calms mind and body
Contraindications: Hamstring or low back injury or strain

***Paschimottanasana* modifications**
- For tight hamstrings: Bend knees to allow the lower back to lengthen
- Use strap around feet to keep elbows bent, shoulders relaxed

Plank
Kid-friendly name: Plank

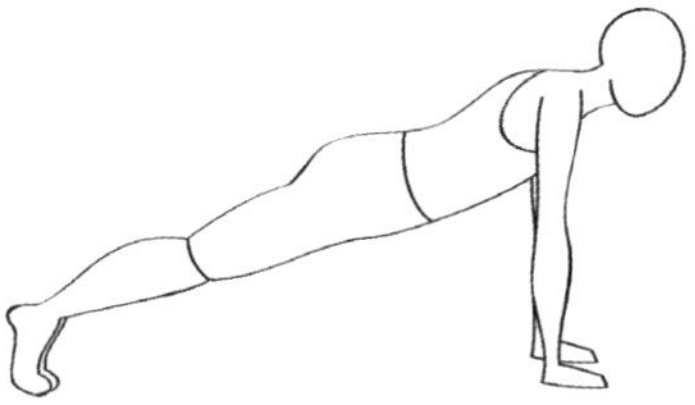

1 Come onto all fours, place wrists directly under shoulders pressing through root knuckles of index finger and thumb while extending through tips of fingers.
2 **Inhale,** shrug shoulders towards ears and then down into "back pockets."
3 **Exhale,** straighten legs and draw lower belly in, until body resembles a plank of wood—straight and long.
4 Tailbone moves towards heels, and gaze a few feet in front of hands.

School-aged children stay in the pose 10–30 seconds. Adolescents can stay 10–60 seconds, depending on strength; children and adolescents may have fun engaging in a friendly contest of who can stay the longest.

Where do you feel it? Arms, shoulders, core
Benefits: Strengthens wrists, arms and back; strengthens core
Contraindications: Wrist injuries

Plank modifications
- For lower back stress: Bend knees to floor (maintaining shoulder and wrist alignment)
- For experienced and strong practitioners: Bend elbows to floor, either clasping hands or extending wrists in line with elbows

Prasarita Padottanasana A
Kid-friendly name: Forward Fold Straddle

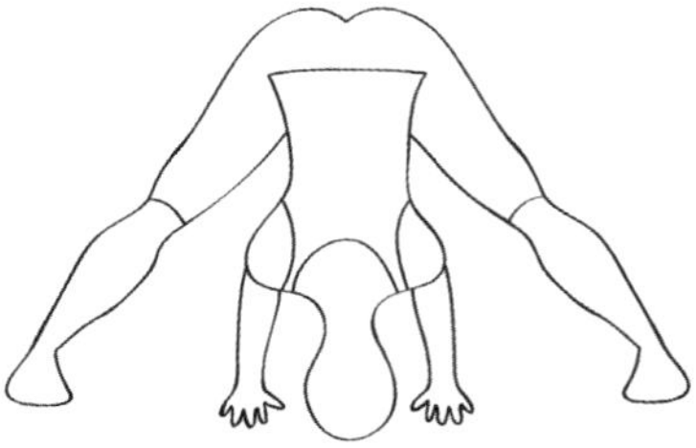

1 Stand in *Tadasana,* Mountain Pose.
2 **Exhale,** place hands on hips and step or jump legs wide.
3 **Inhale,** roll shoulders back, look up toward the ceiling.
4 **Exhale,** hinge at hips to fold forward and place hands on floor.
5 **Inhale,** lengthen torso and release head towards floor, no tension in neck.

School-aged children and adolescents can both stay in the pose for 5–10 breaths, as long as no tightness is felt in the joints (sometimes adolescents are tighter due to growing pains and sports that tighten their muscles. Encourage them to listen to their bodies to determine their capacity, and perhaps only stay 5 breaths).

Where do you feel it? Hamstrings, through length of spine
Benefits: Stretches legs; lengthens spine; relieves overall tension; relieves minor back tension
Contraindications: Lower back injury; certain types of chronic headache, migraine; dizziness or nausea

***Prasarita Padottanasana* modifications**
- For tight hamstrings: Bend knees as deeply as needed to allow hands to rest on floor and allow the head to hang without tension in the neck
- Forward Fold at Bar or Table for lower back injury: Practice pose illustrated in picture below.

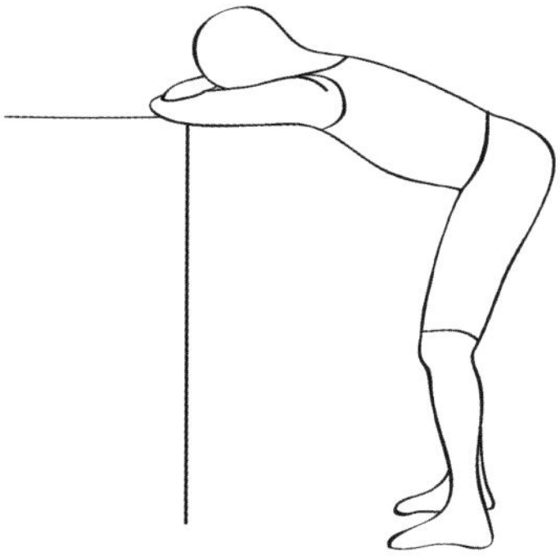

Purvottanasana
Upward Plank Pose
Kid-friendly name: Upward Plank

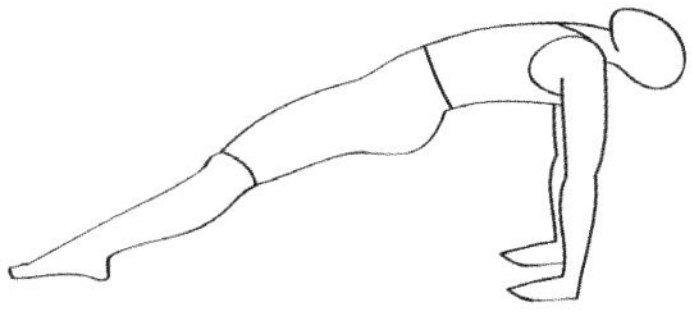

1. Sit on floor, legs extended straight out in front of body.
2. Take arms back, press hands into floor just behind the hips.
3. **Exhale,** draw lower belly in.
4. **Exhale,** extend legs as in picture above.

School-aged children hold the pose for 3–5 breaths. Adolescents can hold 5–10 breaths, or longer (depending on wrist/arm strength, shoulder flexibility, and core strength).

Where do you feel it? Shoulders, chest, back, wrists, buttocks
Benefits: Strengthens core and back; opens chest; invigorates body and mind
Contraindications: Lower back or wrist injury/strain; hypertension

***Purvottanasana* modifications**
- For lower back pain: Set pose up with bent knees/feet on floor before lifting hips, so that body looks like a table top when hips are lifted.
- For mild wrist strain: Place a wedge (high side directly under wrists) under hands before doing pose.

Savasana
Corpse Pose
Kid-friendly name: Relaxation Pose

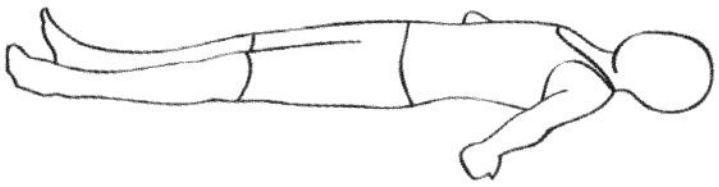

1. Lie supine on floor.
2. **Exhale,** and make fists (thumbs inside fist), flex feet as if standing, and "squinch up" face.
3. Take 2–3 breaths with body tensed like this.
4. **Exhale,** release fists, feet and face.

School-aged children relax in this pose for 5–10 minutes. Whenever possible, allow adolescents a full 10 minutes in Relaxation Pose (as they are often sleep deprived); for this reason, also allow adolescents more time to transition out of this pose.

Where do you feel it? Relaxation throughout body and mind
Benefits: Relaxes and invigorates body; reduces stress; restores multiple body systems
Contraindications: Hypervigilance (such as racing thoughts), psychosis, or trauma.

***Savasana* modifications**

- For scoliosis or large swayback, place several rolled up mats or blankets under knees to lengthen back
- For mild hypervigilance, psychosis or trauma: Leave eyes open or prop back up and cover self with blanket to create a sense of security and comfort
- For moderate to severe hypervigilance, psychosis or trauma: Practice Sa Ta Na Ma mantra instead of any deep relaxation techniques.

Salamba Sarvangasana Variation
Supported Shoulderstand Variation
Kid-friendly name: Candlestick Pose

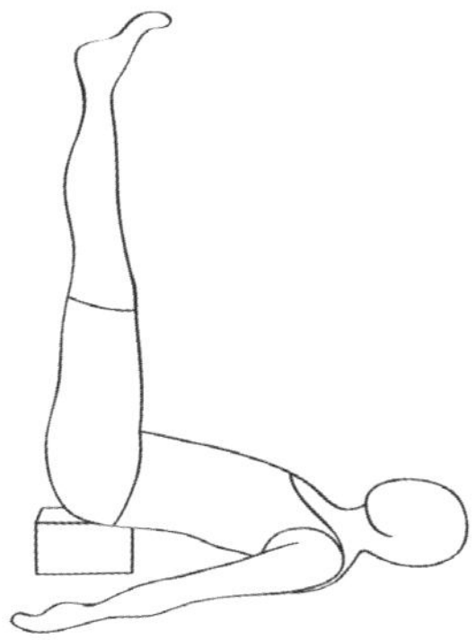

1. Lie on floor with a block nearby.
2. **Inhale** into *Setu Bandha Sarvangasana*, as illustrated but keep arms at sides.
3. **Exhale,** place block under sacrum (lower back just below waistband; feel for a plate of bone that the block can rest underneath).
4. **Inhale,** extend right foot up; **exhale** in place; **inhale,** extend left leg so that big toes touch and heels are slightly separated.

School-aged children can hold the pose for 10–30 seconds. Adolescents can hold 3–5 minutes.

Where do you feel it? Shoulders, chest, back, legs, hips
Benefits: Calms mind; rejuvenates legs
Contraindications: Hypertension; Sacroiliac joint pain/injury

***Salamba Sarvangasana* modifications**

- This pose is itself a modification of Shoulderstand, the classic version of this pose.

Setu Bandha Sarvangasana Vinyasa
Kid-friendly name: Dynamic Bridge

A

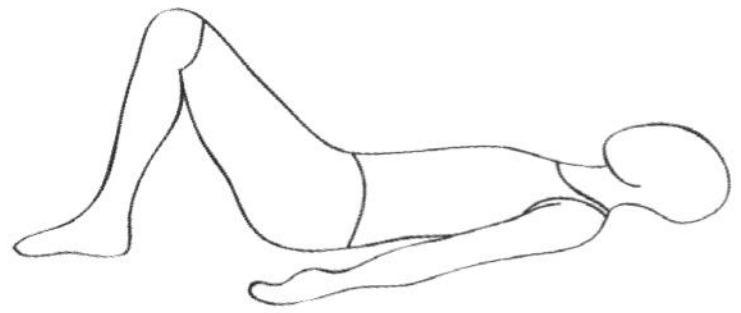

1. Lie on back, knees bent, feet tracking under knees and knees in line with hips.
2. **Exhale,** press through feet and arms.

B

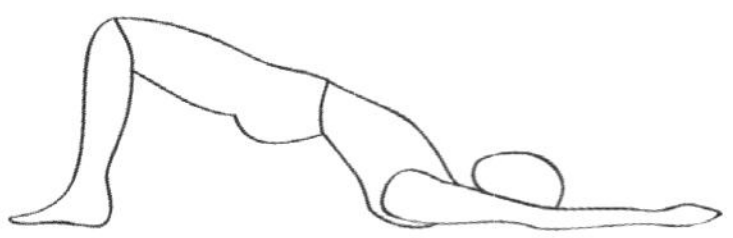

3. **Inhale,** lift arms (overhead on the floor) and hips, as shown in step B.
4. **Exhale,** and bring hips and arms back down, as in step A.

School-aged children repeat up to 5 times. Adolescents repeat 5– 10 times.

Where do you feel it? Shoulders, chest, legs, hips
Benefits: Energizes body and mind (very good for depression); strengthens legs; increases blood flow in head, neck and shoulders; good for those who suffer from chronic headache
Contraindications: Sacroiliac joint, hip or ankle pain/injury

Dynamic Bridge modifications

- For those with minor back issues: Lift hips slightly (rather than to full range of motion).

Sucirandhrasana
Kid-friendly name: Eye-of-the-Needle

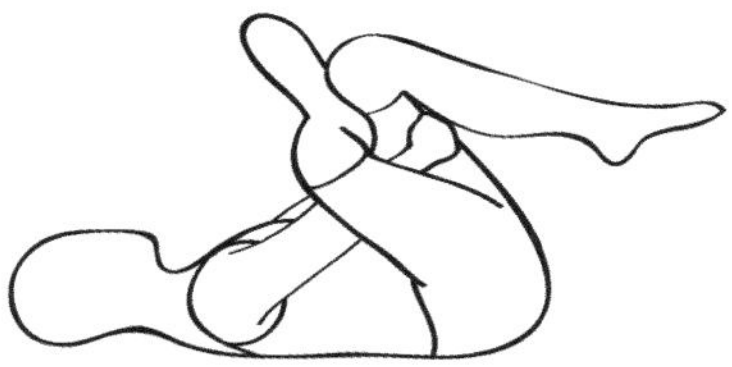

1. Lie supine on floor, knees bent.
2. Cross right ankle over left knee.
3. **Exhale,** thread right hand between legs and grab left leg with both hands on either side of leg.
4. **Inhale,** rest head on floor (if it came up while clasping the hands behind the left leg) and roll shoulders back to the floor.
5. If flexible, draw left leg towards chest and press right knee away from body to increase the stretch in the right outer hip.
6. Repeat on other side for equal number of breaths or counts.

School-aged children hold for 5–10 breaths. Adolescents can hold 10–20 breaths.

Where do you feel it? Outer hip of leg that's bent out to the side; lower back stretch
Benefits: Increases hip flexibility; releases tension in lower back and outer hip and leg (very good for runners)
Contraindications: diarrhea; major sacroiliac issues

***Sucirandhrasana* modifications**

- For tight hips: Keep left foot on floor and enjoy stretch in outer right hip.

Sukhasana
Simple Sitting Pose
Kid-friendly name: Criss-Cross Apple Sauce

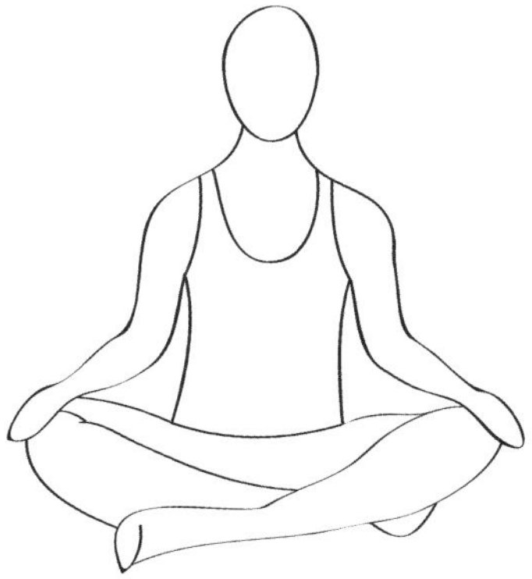

1. Sit on floor and cross legs.
2. Allow hands to rest on legs wherever they feel comfortable.
3. **Inhale,** shrug shoulders up and back.
4. **Exhale,** rock gently from side to side until both sitting bones feel equally grounded.
5. Close eyes if mind feels scattered; keep eyes open if feeling sleepy.

School-aged children hold the pose for 5–10 breaths. Adolescents hold for 10 breaths or longer.

Where do you feel it? Shoulders, chest, spine
Benefits: Calms and invigorates body and mind; increases hip flexibility; increases concentration and focus

Contraindications: Lower back injury/strain

***Sukhasana* modifications**
- For lower back pain: Sit on a block, blanket or chair
- For tight knees: Support knee that's off floor with a prop
- For tight ankles: Uncross ankles

Sukhasana Twist
Kid-friendly name: Seated Twist

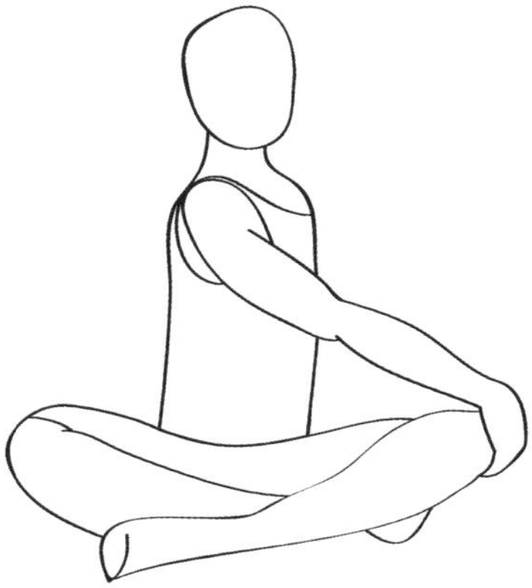

1 Sit in *Sukhasana*, Simple Sitting Pose.
2 **Inhale,** shrug shoulders up and back.
3 **Exhale,** turn towards right knee, placing left hand on right knee.
4 **Inhale,** lengthen through spine.
5 **Exhale,** turn lower belly towards back wall.
6 **Inhale,** lengthen through spine.
7 **Exhale,** twist mid-belly towards back wall.
8 **Inhale,** re-lengthen spine.
9 **Exhale,** turn chest and chin to look over right shoulder (if comfortable).
10 Repeat on other side for equal number of breaths or counts.

School-aged children hold the pose for 5 – 10 breaths. Adolescents hold for 10 breaths or longer.

Where do you feel it? Shoulders, chest, spine
Benefits: Invigorates body and mind; relieves tension in back; increases hip flexibility
Contraindications: Lower back injury/strain; pregnancy

***Sukhasana Twist* modifications**
- For lower back pain: Sit on a block, blanket or chair

Supported (Passive) Backbend
Kid-friendly name: Supported Backbend

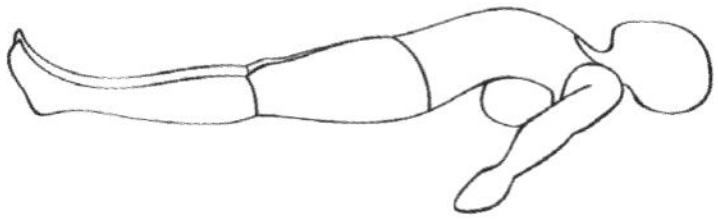

1 Sit on the floor with legs extended and place a tightly rolled mat or firm blanket behind the back perpendicular to the spine.
2 **Exhale,** lie down over rolled mat or blanket — place it just above the lower back and below the shoulder blades.
3 **Inhale,** roll shoulders back.
4 **Exhale,** lengthen the torso.

School-aged children and adolescents can stay in the version of this pose that best supports their back for up to 5 minutes.

Where do you feel it? Chest, deeper breathing, stiller mind
Benefits: Deeply restorative—relieves stress, teaches a deep state of relaxation and surrender

Contraindications: Significant lordosis (swayback, or lower back curvature) or scoliosis; hypervigilance, active psychosis or trauma (the stillness and surrender of this pose is inadvisable for those with the above-mentioned symptoms, and causes/increases racing thoughts, decreased self-esteem, and other negative symptoms)

Supported Backbend modifications

- For those with significant lordosis (swayback) or scoliosis, place several rolled mats or blankets under knees to decrease lower back curve
- Support neck with prop underneath head (ensure that the prop is not greater in height than the prop under the back)
- For psychosis, hypervigilance or trauma: Practice Sa Ta Na Ma mantra instead

Supta Padangusthasana
Kid-friendly name: Reclining Big Toe Pose

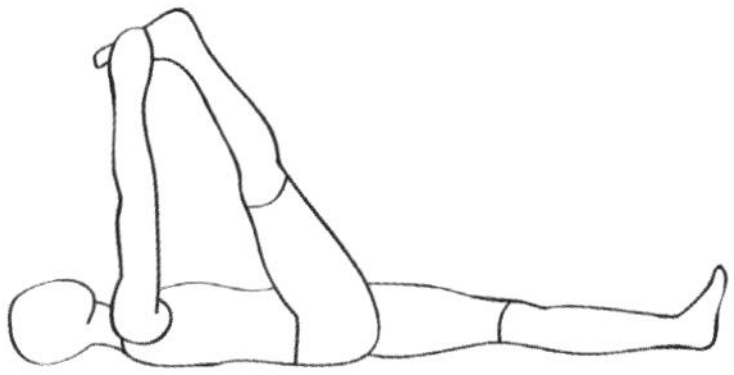

1 Lie on floor, knees bent.
2 **Inhale,** extend right leg up, sole of foot facing ceiling.
3 **Exhale,** loop strap around right foot or take big right toe with first two fingers ("peace" fingers).
4 **Inhale,** extend right leg so that the stretch is felt in the *belly* (middle) of the right hamstring.
5 For those who need more stretch, extend left leg straight on floor while digging left heel into floor to maintain energy and awareness in left leg.
6 Repeat on other side for equal number of breaths or counts.

School-aged children and adolescents can hold for the pose for 5–10 breaths.

Where do you feel it? Middle of hamstring muscles
Benefits: Increases hip and hamstring flexibility; releases tension in lower back and outer hip and leg (very good for runners and athletes who run a lot in their sports, e.g. soccer)
Contraindications: Hamstring injury

***Supta Padangusthasana* modifications**

- For tight hamstrings or back: Grab back of knee of extended leg with both hands; Keep "bottom" leg bent
- For very flexible individuals: Be sure to maintain an isometric stretch, meaning resist the stretch so that the sensation is felt in the belly of the hamstring muscle, and not down towards the knee or up towards the sitting bone

Surya Namaskar
Kid-Friendly Name: Sun Salutation

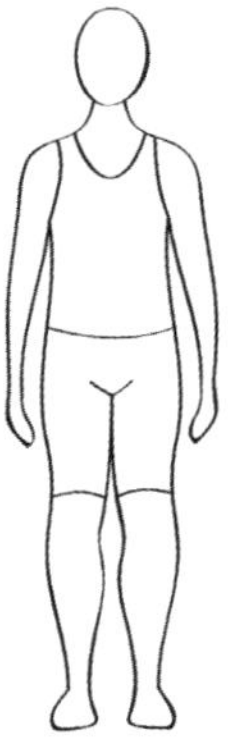

1 Exhale

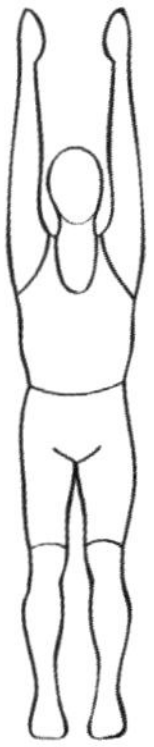

2 Inhale

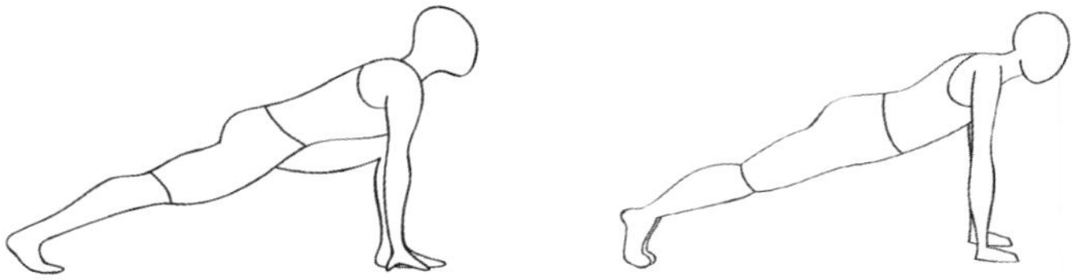

3 Exhale, step 1 foot back and then the other

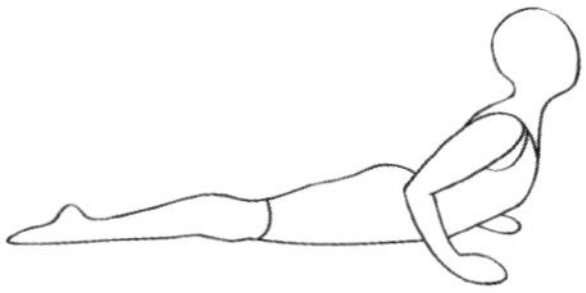

4 Inhale into Cobra

OR

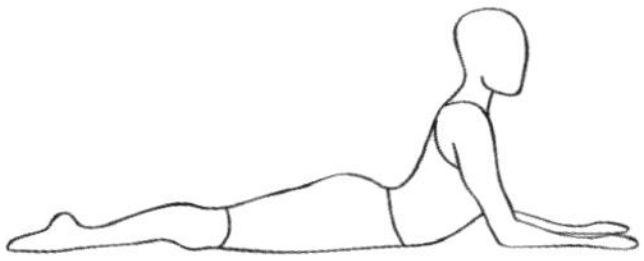

Sphinx (for back injury or pain)

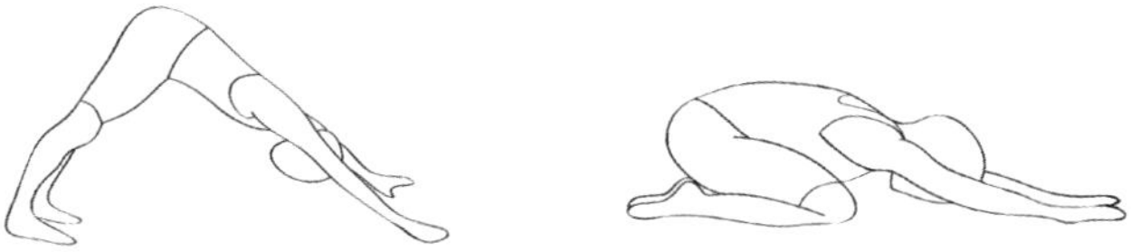

5 Exhale into Downward Dog OR Rock Pose (for a more calming practice)

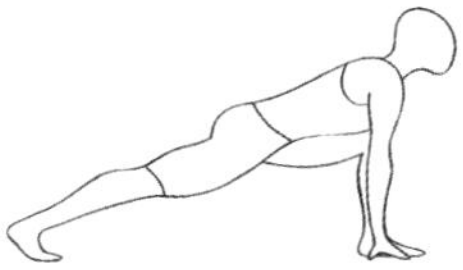

6 Exhale

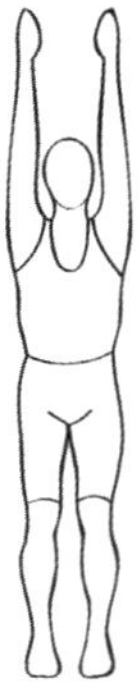

7 Inhale

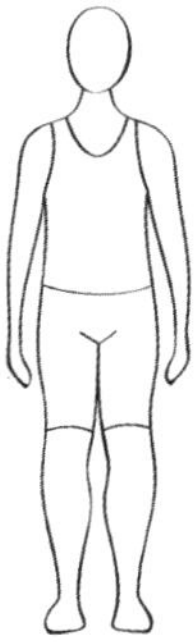

8 Exhale

Tadasana
Mountain Pose
Kid-friendly name: Mountain Pose

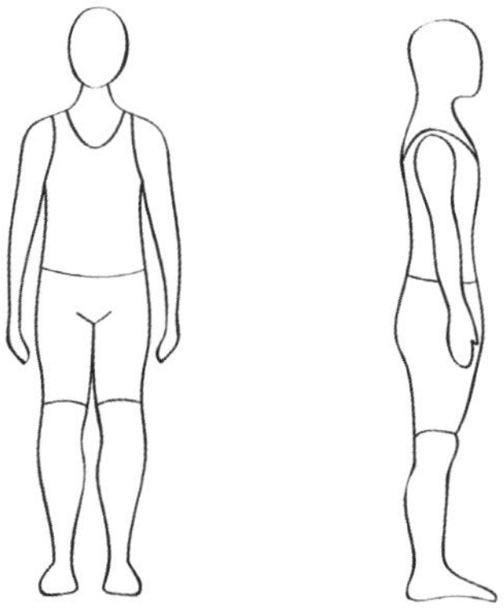

1. Stand with feet hip distance apart.
2. **Inhale,** lift toes.
3. **Exhale,** spread toes like fan on floor (without gripping).
4. **Inhale,** shrug shoulders up towards ears and back.
5. **Exhale,** drop shoulders down as if into back pockets.
6. **Inhale,** extend the spine like the stalk of a sunflower reaching towards the sun.
7. **Exhale,** feel the feet ground downwards, as if roots were growing down into the ground as far down as your head reaches above it.

School-aged children hold the pose for 5–10 breaths. Adolescents can hold 10–20 breaths, depending on ability to focus in the present moment.

Where do you feel it? Throughout body and mind
Benefits: Activates awareness and muscle engagement in legs, core and throughout body; calms mind through focus and attention to body sensations and alignment

***Tadasana* modifications**

- For those who can't stand, sit in a chair with same alignment instructions, use sitting bones as foundation.

Upavistha Konasana
Wide-Angled Seated Pose
Kid-friendly name: Wide Angle Pose

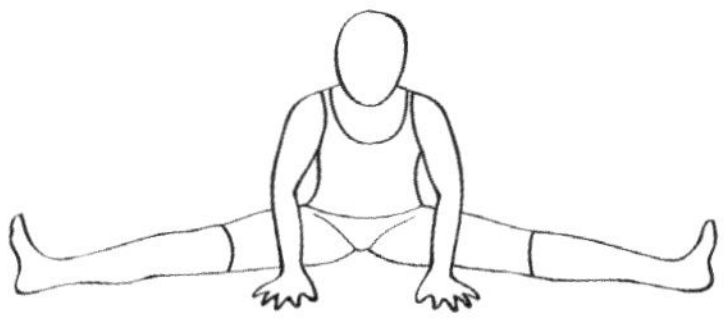

1. Sit in *Sukhasana,* Simple Sitting Pose.
2. **Inhale,** extend legs in front of you at a wide angle and roll shoulders up and back.
3. **Exhale,** reach chest forward and down; step hands out in front on the floor.
4. **Inhale,** lengthen through spine.
5. **Exhale,** sitting bones sink into the floor.

School-aged children hold the pose for 5–10 breaths; adolescents hold for 10 breaths or longer.

Where do you feel it? Hamstrings, back, hips, calves
Benefits: Invigorates body and mind; relieves tension in back; increases hip and hamstring flexibility
Contraindications: Hamstring, hip or lower back injury/strain

***Upavistha Konasana* modifications**

- For lower back or hamstring issues: Sit on a block or blanket and/or bend knees, digging heels into floor, big toes facing straight up.

Utthita Parsvakonasana
Extended Side Angle Pose
Kid-friendly name: Side Angle Pose

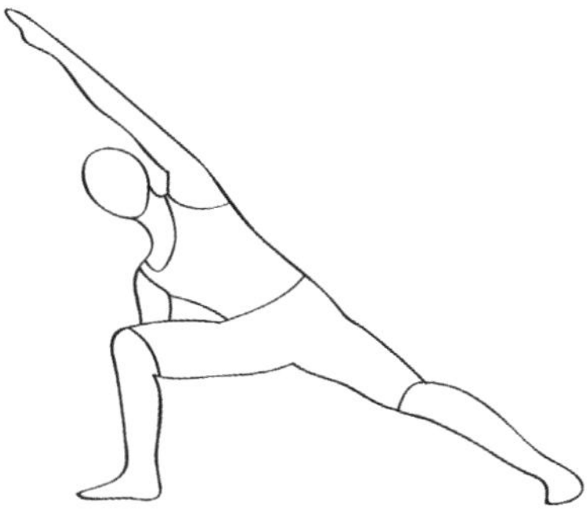

1 Stand in *Tadasana*, Mountain Pose.
2 **Exhale,** step or jump legs as wide as wrists when arms are extended.
3 **Inhale,** roll shoulders back, and extend arms out to sides.
4 **Exhale,** turn toes towards right, bend right knee directly over right ankle, and place right elbow on right thigh OR place right finger tips on block or floor on outside of right ankle (as in picture above).
5 **Inhale,** spin torso towards ceiling, look up beyond right armpit (as long as no neck strain is felt), and extend equally through right arm and right leg/foot.
6 **Exhale,** press right knee into right arm or until right knee faces in same direction as toes.
7 Repeat on other side for equal number of breaths or counts.

School-aged children hold each side of the pose for 5–10 breaths. Adolescents hold each side for 10 or more breaths, depending on strength.

Where do you feel it? Legs, arms, hips, ribs/side waist and shoulders
Benefits: Strengthens and stretches legs; lengthens spine; energizes body and mind
Contraindications: Lower back injury; certain types of chronic headache, migraine; dizziness or nausea

Utthita Parsvakonasana **modifications**

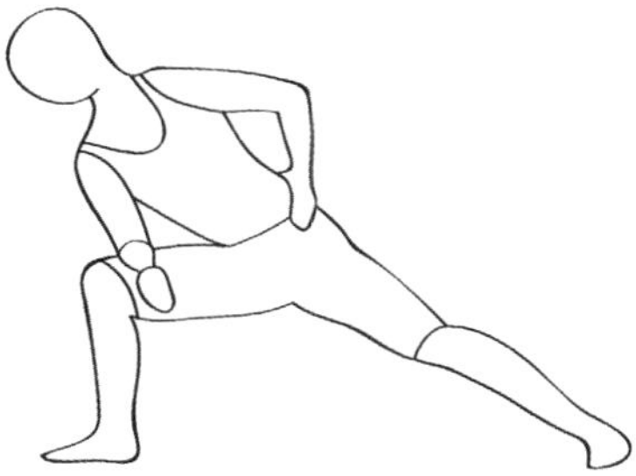

- For tight hamstrings or hips: Place elbow on leg as in picture above
- For tight shoulders or neck: Place "top" hand on hip instead
- For stiff neck: Look directly forward (or down) rather than up towards ceiling

Utthita Trikonasana
Extended Triangle Pose
Kid-friendly name: Triangle Pose

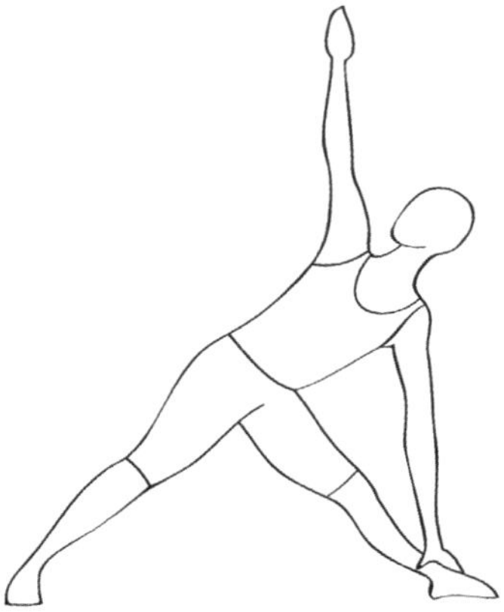

1 Stand in *Tadasana*, Mountain Pose.
2 **Exhale,** step or jump legs apart as wide as wrists when arms are extended.
3 **Inhale,** roll shoulders back, and extend arms out to sides.

4 **Exhale,** reach right hand in direction of right toes (as if fencing) and then let right hand drop onto right leg either above or below the knee while still keeping spine long and shoulders relaxed.
5 **Inhale,** twist torso towards ceiling, extend right hand straight up towards ceiling.
6 **Exhale,** press outer edge of right foot down while extending tailbone towards right heel.
7 Repeat on other side for equal number of breaths or counts.

School-aged children hold each side of the pose for 5–10 breaths. Adolescents hold each side for 10 or more breaths, depending on strength and flexibility.

Where do you feel it? Legs, spine, arms, hips, ribs/side waist and shoulders
Benefits: Strengthens and stretches legs; lengthens spine; energizes body and mind
Contraindications: Lower back injury; certain types of chronic headache, migraine; dizziness or nausea

***Utthita Trikonasana* modifications**

- For tight hamstrings or hips: Place hand on a block, or higher up the leg than shown in the picture
- For tight shoulders or neck: Place "top" hand on hip instead
- For stiff neck: Look directly forward (or down) rather than up towards ceiling

Viparita Karani
Legs-Up-the-Wall Pose
Kid-friendly name: Legs-Up-the-Wall Pose

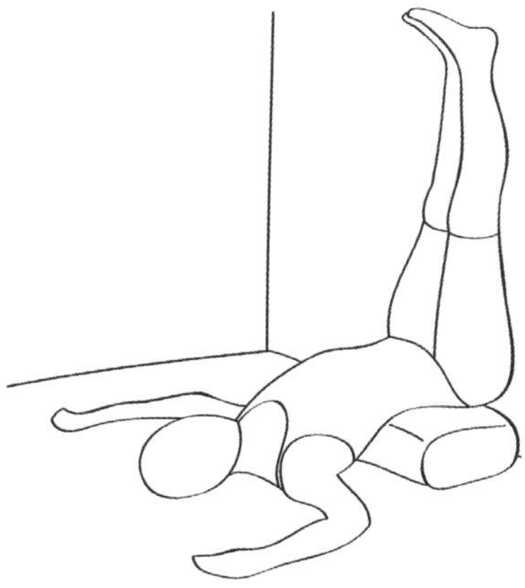

1 Sit on floor next to a wall (*optional:* sit on a stack of blankets so that hips will be elevated while in the pose as shown in the picture).
2 Lean back, swivel hips so the buttocks are touching the wall and extend legs up the wall.
3 Place arms in whatever position is most comfortable: on the belly, at the sides of the body or up above the head on the floor.

For beginners to this pose: stay in it for 1–3 minutes. For children and adolescents who have practiced this pose with some degree of frequency, stay 5 minutes or longer.

Where do you feel it? Shoulders, chest, spine, legs
Benefits: Calms body and mind; relaxes and invigorates legs; relieves tension in shoulders, head and neck; can relieve some types of chronic headache (individual preference)
Contraindications: Hypervigilance; trauma (individual preference)
Note: *Viparita Karani* and *Salamba Sarvangasana* variation are very similar poses. *Salamba Sarvangasana* variation is an active restorative pose as the legs, belly and the lower half of the body are engaged. Viparita Karani, on the other hand, is most definitely a restorative pose, in which most muscles are relaxed. But they are both restorative inversions, and aid digestion, sleep and circulation.

***Viparita Karani* modifications**

- For tight hamstrings: adjust blankets slightly away from wall so that hips are also a small distance from the wall, allowing legs to rest naturally on wall
- For uncomfortable tingling in legs: stay a shorter time in pose OR bend knees and bring soles of the feet together
- For mild hypervigilance or trauma: Try doing it flat on the floor, rather than on blankets so that the head is in line (and not lower than) the rest of the torso
- For moderate to severe hypervigilance or trauma: Avoid this pose

Virabhadrasana I
Warrior Pose I
Kid-friendly name: Peaceful Warrior Pose I

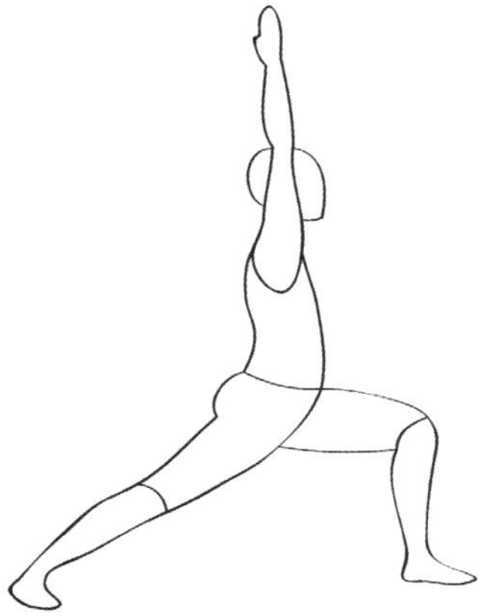

1. Stand in *Tadasana,* Mountain Pose.
2. **Exhale,** step left foot back; angle foot so that heel touches floor; bend right knee directly over right ankle as in a lunge.
3. **Inhale,** extend arms upwards.
4. **Exhale,** roll shoulders back to release tension in the neck and shoulders.
5. **Inhale,** lengthen down through back leg and up through spine.
6. **Exhale,** press outer edge of left foot down while extending tailbone towards right heel.
7. Repeat on other side for equal number of breaths or counts.

School-aged children hold each side of the pose for 5 – 10 breaths. Adolescents hold each side 10 or more breaths, depending on strength and flexibility.

Where do you feel it? Legs, spine, arms, hips and shoulders
Benefits: Strengthens and stretches legs; lengthens spine; energizes body and mind
Contraindications: High blood pressure or heart problems

***Virabhadrasana I* modifications**
- Shorten stance for lower back, knee or hip injury/strain
- For shoulder problems: keep hands & arms shoulder distance (don't bring hands together)
- For neck problems: look forward and not up at hands

Virabhadrasana II
Warrior Pose II
Kid-friendly name: Peaceful Warrior Pose II

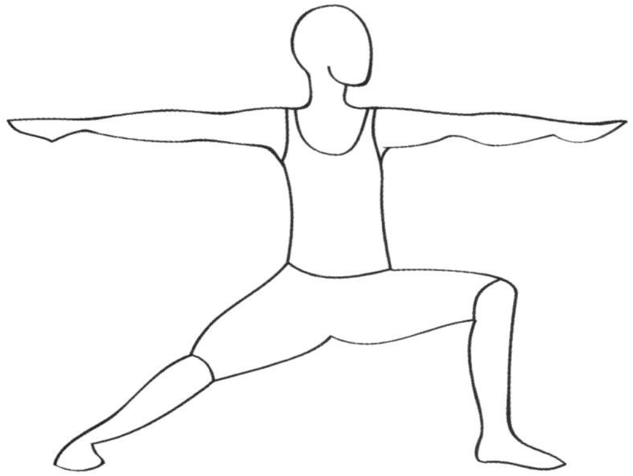

1. Stand in *Tadasana,* Mountain Pose.
2. **Exhale,** step or jump legs as wide as wrists when arms are extended.
3. **Inhale,** roll shoulders back, and extend arms out to sides.
4. **Exhale,** bend right knee directly over right ankle.
5. **Inhale,** lengthen through spine and extend equally through left arm.
6. **Exhale,** press outer edge of right foot down while extending tailbone towards right heel.
7. Repeat on other side for equal number of breaths or counts.

School-aged children hold each side of the pose for 5–10 breaths. Adolescents hold each side for 10 or more breaths, depending on strength and flexibility.

Where do you feel it? Legs, spine, arms, hips and shoulders
Benefits: Strengthens and stretches legs; lengthens spine; energizes body and mind
Contraindications: Knee or hip injury/strain

***Virabhadrasana II* modifications**
- Shorten stance for lower back, knee or hip injury/strain
- For shoulder or neck strain: Place hands on hips

Vrksasana
Tree Pose
Kid-friendly name: Tree Pose

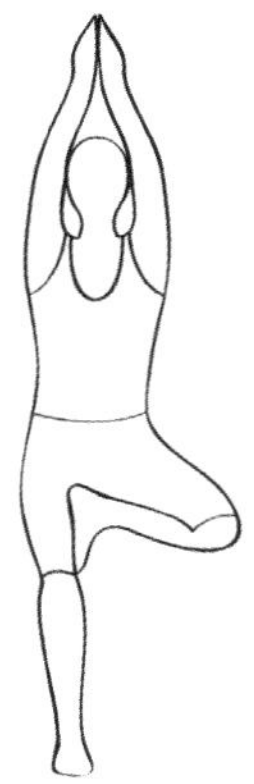

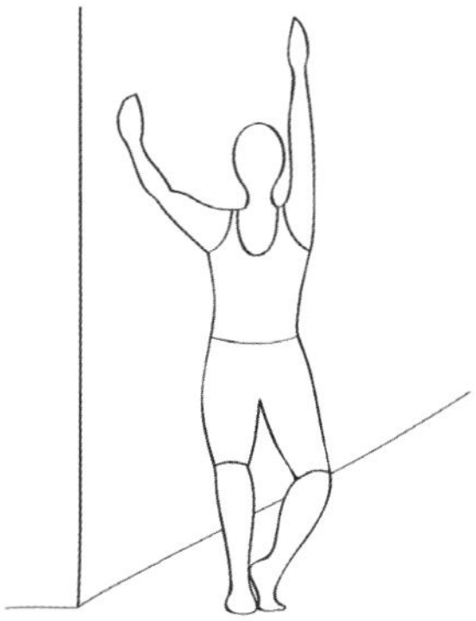

1. Stand in *Tadasana*, Mountain Pose.
2. **Exhale,** feel the feet ground downwards, as if roots were growing down into the ground as far down as your head reaches above it, and place hands on hips.
3. As a challenge and if balance is OK, inhale and extend arms overhead as in Figure A above.
4. Exhale.

School-aged children hold 5–10 breaths. Adolescents can hold 10–20 breaths, depending on ability to focus in the present moment.

Where do you feel it? Focused mind; arm stretched
Benefits: Cultivates balance; engages muscles in legs, core; stretches arms; calms mind through act of balancing

Contraindications: Hip, knee, ankle injuries/major strain

***Vrksasana* modifications**

- For those with balance issues: Put hand on wall and/or put bent-knee big toe on floor, as in Figure B above.

Windshield Wipers
Kid-friendly name: Windshield Wipers Pose

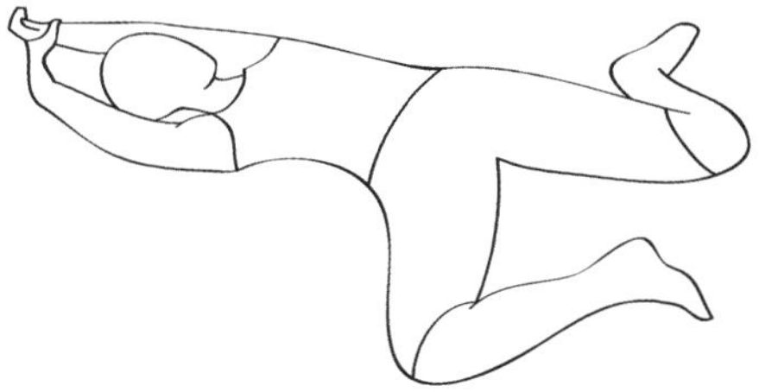

1. Lie supine on the floor, knees bent, feet turned out like "duck feet".
2. **Exhale,** drop both knees to the left so that right knee aligns directly in line with right. hip (left knee bent to the left as shown in the picture).
3. **Inhale,** extend arms above head on the floor.
4. **Exhale,** feel stretch intensify in lower belly and/or upper, inner right leg.
5. **Inhale,** reach through arms (to increase stretch, take right wrist with left hand).
6. **Exhale,** extend through right knee.
7. Repeat on other side for equal number of breaths or counts.

School-aged children hold each side of the pose for 5–10 breaths; adolescents hold each side for 10 or more breaths, depending on flexibility.

Where do you feel it? Lower belly, hip of extended knee, upper leg
Benefits: Strengthens and stretches legs; lengthens spine; energizes body and mind
Contraindications: Psoas or knee injury

Windshield Wiper Modifications

- For psoas or knee issues: avoid this pose
- For a greater stretch: grab wrist of the knee that is extending downward and pull on wrist while exhaling

Visualizations and relaxation exercises

Five-Minute Vacation

Can be used with any age group.

- Lie down, close your eyes and relax. If feeling anxious or restless, ball up fists, feet and face for three breaths. Exhale and release fists, feet and face.
- Imagine a special place you'd like to go on vacation. It could be a place you've been to before, a place you've always wanted to go or a place from your imagination. In this place, you feel totally yourself and completely relaxed.
- Ring bell: As the bell rings, imagine you're travelling to that place now.
- Look around you. What do you see? Are you inside or outside? Is it day or night? Notice all the objects, or the things in nature. Maybe you find yourself on a deserted beach, or a high mountain top, or a favorite amusement park.
- What do you hear? Do you hear music? The sounds of nature? People laughing?
- What do you smell in your vacation spot? Can you smell beautiful flowers? Or the smell of salty air? Maybe your favorite food is cooking somewhere close by...
- Notice if you're alone, or if you'd invite family, friends or pets who make you feel totally yourself, completely relaxed. Whatever is right for you, imagine that.
- Now notice how you feel when you're in this special place where you're totally yourself, completely relaxed. Just rest, knowing there's nowhere to go, nothing to be. Everything is ok.

The yoga therapist can continue this visualization for as long as the time allotted, or until students begin to stir. Make sure to bring students out of this slowly and mindfully.

Green Breath Meditation

This is best for adolescents but some school-aged children also love this practice.

- Lie down, close your eyes and relax. If feeling anxious or restless, ball up fists, feet and face for three breaths. Exhale and release fists, feet and face.
- Notice your breath coming in and going out. Inhale, feel the opening, expansive, lengthening qualities of inhalation. Exhale, feel the dropping, rooting, grounding qualities of exhalation.
- As you breathe, imagine all the trees outside this room that you can't see. Even though you can't see them, as you breathe in you're breathing in the oxygen they give off. As you exhale, you offer the carbon dioxide you breathe out.
- Now imagine a park or wooded area you like. Imagine all the trees, grasses and plants in that area. Imagine that as you inhale, you're breathing in the oxygen from all those trees, grasses and plants. As you exhale, you're feeding them. Even when you're not aware of it, this supportive, harmonious relationship is going on all the time.
- Enjoy this exchange. If you can, expand your awareness to the whole city. As you inhale, breathe in all the oxygen from every tree and plant in the city. As you exhale, give back to the trees and plants.

The yoga therapist can continue this visualization for as long as the time allotted, or until students begin to stir. Facilitate a slow and mindful transition from relaxing to sitting up.

Sa Ta Na Ma Mantra

This is best for adolescents but some school-aged children may also enjoy it.

- Sit up tall, but relaxed. Notice the breath coming in and going out.
- Bring thumbs and index fingers together and say "Sa"

- Bring thumbs and middle fingers together and say "Ta"
- Bring thumbs and ring fingers together and say "Na"
- Bring thumbs and pinkie fingers together and say "Ma"
- Repeat 5–10 times

Try slowing the last few repetitions down even further, and notice what happens to the speed of your thoughts and your state of mind.

Yoga Nidra (best for School-aged children and adolescents)

There are many versions of *Yoga Nidra* available for purchase. However, if working with school-aged children or younger, it's important to find a version that is kid-friendly. Follow this link for a kid-tested version that we use at Children's Hospital Colorado: http://www.childrenscolorado.org/departments/psych/programs/creative-arts-therapy/yoga-therapy, and click at the bottom of the page where it says "Listen to a Yoga Nidra relaxation recording."

References

ADD Treatment Center (2005) Can ADHD be prevented in early intervention? [online] Available from: http://www.addtreatmentcenters.com/framefiles/articles/Can%20ADHD%20be%20Prevented%20by%20Early%20Intervention.html [Accessed 26 September 2014].

APA, (2015) Citations and abstracts; Motivation for dieting: Drive for thinness different than objective thinness. [online]. Available at http://psycnet.apa.org/?&fa=main.doiLanding&doi=10.1037/a0018398 [Accessed 4 Mar 2015].

American Physical Therapy Association, (2003) *The Guide to Physical Therapist Practice, Second Edition.* Alexandria: American Physical Therapy Association.

American Foundation for Suicide Prevention (2014) Risk factors and warning signs. [online] Available from: https://www.afsp.org/preventing-suicide/risk-factors-and-warning-signs [Accessed 29 August 2014].

American Psychiatric Publishing (2013) Feeding and Eating Disorders. *Diagnostic and Statistical Manual of Mental Disorders* (DSM-5) [online] Available from: http://www.dsm5.org/documents/eatingdisordersfactsheet.pdf [Accessed 13 May 2014].

American Psychiatric Publishing (2013) Posttraumatic Stress Disorder. [online] Available from: http://www.dsm5.org/Documents/PTSDSpringer sheet.pdf [Accessed 5 June 2014].

Baliki, M.N., Geha, P.Y., Apkarian, A.V. & Chialvo, D.R. (2008) Beyond feeling: chronic pain hurts the brain, disrupting the default-mode network dynamics. *The Journal of Neuroscience.* 28 (6). p.1398–1403.

Bangalore, N.G. & Varambally, S. (2012) Yoga therapy for schizophrenia. *International Journal of Yoga.* 5 (2). p.85–91.

Beaudette, R. & Harhen, P. (2008) TEACCH (Treatment and Education of Autistic and Communication-Handicapped Children). [online] Available from: http://www.readbag.com/scituatespedpac-presentations-teacch.

Bennett, S.M., Weintraub, A. & Khalsa, S.B.S. (2008) Initial evaluation of the LifeForce yoga program as a therapeutic intervention for depression. *International Association of Yoga Therapy.* 18. p.49–57.

Bettelheim, B. (1982) Freud and the Soul. [online] Available from: https://www.newyorker.com/archive/1982/03/01/1982_03_01_052 [Accessed 1 November 2013].

Birchwood, M. & MacMillan, F. (1993) Early intervention in schizophrenia. *Australia and New Zealand Journal of Psychiatry.* 27 (3). p.374–378.

Birdee, G.S. Yeh, G.Y., Wayne, P.M., Phillips, R.S., Davis, R.B., & Gardiner, P. (2009) Clinical applications of yoga for the pediatric population: a systematic review. *Academic Pediatrics.* 9 (4). p.212–220.

Booth, R. (2014) Mindfulness therapy comes at a high price for some, say experts. [online] Available from: http://www.theguardian.com/society/2014/aug/25/mental-health-meditation/print [Accessed 25 August 2014].

Boudette, R. (2006) Question & answer: yoga in the treatment of disordered eating and body image disturbance. How can the practice of yoga be helpful in recovery from an eating disorder? *Eating Disorders.* 14. p.167–170.

Bowen Theory (2008) *Bowen Theory.* [online] Available from: http://www.thebowencenter.org/pages/theory.html [Accessed 6 December 2013].

Brach, T. (2003) *Radical Acceptance: Embracing Your Life with the Heart of a Buddha.* New York: Bantam Books.

Briere, J. N. (1992) *Child Abuse Trauma: Theory and Treatment of the Lasting Effects.* Newbury Park: Sage Publications.

Broderick, P.C. & Metz, S. (2009) Learning to BREATHE: a pilot trial of a mindfulness curriculum for adolescents. *Advances in School Mental Health Promotion.* 2 (1). p.35–36.

Broome, M.R., Woolley, J.B., Tabraham, P., Johns, L.C., Bramon, E., Murrary, G.K., Pariante, C., McGuire, P.K., & Murray, R.M. (2005) What causes the onset of psychosis? *Schizophrenia Research.* 79 (1). p.23–34.

Bryan, L.C. & Gast, D.L. (2000) Teaching on-task and on-schedule behaviors to high-functioning children with autism via picture activity schedules. *Journal of Autism and Developmental Disorders.* 30 (6). p.553–567.

Cabral, P., Meyer, H.B. & Ames, D. (2011) Effectiveness of yoga therapy as a complementary treatment for major psychiatric disorders: a meta-analysis. *Primary Companion for CNS Disorders.* 13 (4), [online] Available from: http://www.ncbi.nlm.nih.gov/pmc/articles/PMC3219516 [Accessed 7 August 2014].

Carei, T.R., Fyfe-Johnson, A.L., Breuner, C.C. & Brown, M.A. (2010) Randomized controlled clinical trial of yoga in the treatment of eating disorders. *Journal of Adolescent Health.* 46. p.346–351.

Centers for Disease Control and Prevention (2014) Attention-Deficit/Hyperactivity Disorder: Symptoms and Diagnosis. [online] Available from: http://www.cdc.gov/ncbddd/adhd/diagnosis.html [Accessed 26 September 2014].

Centers for Disease Control and Prevention (2014) CDC estimates 1 in 68 children has been identified with autism spectrum disorder. [online] Available from: http://www.cdc.gov/media/releases/2014/p0327-autism-spectrum-disorder.html [Accessed 8 October 2014].

Centers for Disease Control and Prevention (2014) Suicide prevention: youth suicide. [online] Available from: http://www.cdc.gov/violenceprevention/pub/youth_suicide.html [Accessed 28 August 2014].

Chapman, A.L., Gratz, K.L. & Turner, B.J. (2014) Risk-related and protective correlates of nonsuicidal self-injury and co-occurring suicide attempts among incarcerated women. *Suicide Life-Threatening Behavior.* 44 (2). p.139–154.

Cherry, K. (2014) Implicit and explicit memory: two types of long-term memory. [online] Available from: http://psychology.about.com/od/memory/a/implicit-and-explicit-memory.htm [Accessed 21 July 2014].

Cherry, K. (2014) What is mania? [online] Available from: http://psychology.about.com/od/mindex/g/mania [Accessed 10 September 2014].

Child Mind Institute (2014) FAQs about autism. [online] Available from: http://www.childmind.org/en/autism-faqs/ [Accessed 8 October 2014].

Cohen, S. & Schwarz, A (2013) A.D.H.D. Seen in 11% of U.S. Children as Diagnoses Rise [online] Available from: http://www.nytimes.com/2013/04/01/health/more-diagnoses-of-hyperactivity-causing-concern.html?pagewanted=all&_r=1& [Accessed 12 September 2014].

Cook, A., Spinazzola, J., Ford, J., Lanktree, C., Blaustein, M., Cloitre, M., DeRosa, R., Hubbard, R., Kagan, R., Liautaud, J., Mallah, K., Olafson, E., & van der Kolk, B. (2005) Complex trauma in children and adolescents. *Psychiatric Annals.* 35 (5). p.390–398.

Cook-Cottone, C., Beck, M., & Kane, L. (2008) Manualized group treatment of eating disorders: attunement in mind, body, and relationship. *Journal for Specialists in Group Work.* 33 (1). p. 61–83.

da Silva. T.L., Ravidran, L.N. & Ravidran. A.V. (2009) Yoga in the treatment of mood and anxiety disorders: a review. *Asian Journal of Psychiatry.* 2. p.6–16.

Daubenmier, J.J. (2005) The relationship of yoga, body awareness, and body responsiveness to self-objectification and disordered eating. *Psychology of Women Quarterly.* 29. pp. 207–219.

Delaney, K., & Anthis, K., (2010) Is women's participation in different types of yoga classes associated with different levels of body awareness and body satisfaction? *International Journal of Yoga Therapy.* 20. p. 28-37.

Dittman, K.A., & Freedman, M.R. (2009) Body awareness, eating attitudes and spiritual beliefs of women practicing yoga. *Eating Disorders,* 17 (4). p. 273–92.

Duraiswamy, G., Thirthalli, J., Nagendra, H.R. & Gangadhar, B.N. (2007) Yoga therapy as an add-on treatment in the management of patients with schizophrenia: a randomized controlled trial. *Acta Psychiatrica Scandanavica.* 116. p.226–232.

Ehrenreich, J.G., Goldstein, C.M., Wright, L.R. & Barlow, D.H. (2009) Development of a unified protocol for the treatment of emotional disorders in youth. *Child and Family Behavior Therapy.* 31 (1). p. 20–37.

Emerson, D. & Hopper, E. (2011) *Overcoming Trauma through Yoga: Reclaiming Your Body*. Berkeley: North Atlantic Books.

Epstein, M. (1995) *Thoughts Without a Thinker: Psychotherapy from a Buddhist Perspective*. New York: Basic Books.

Evans, S., Moieni, M., Sternlieg, B., Tsao, J.C.I., & Zeltzer, L. (2012) Yoga for youth: the UCLA Pediatric Pain Program Model. *Holistic Nursing Practice.* 26 (5). p.262–271.

Ezraty, M. (2007) Defining Vinyasa. [online] Available from: http://www.yogajournal.com/article/teach/defining-vinyasa/ [Accessed 20 September 2014].

Farchione, T.J., Fairholme, C.P., Ellard, K.K., Boisseau, C.L., Thompson-Hollands, J., Carl, J.R., Gallagher, M.W., & Barlow, D.H. (2012) Unified protocol for transdiagnostic treatment of emotional disorders: a randomized controlled trial. *Behavior Therapy.* 43 (3). p.666–678.

Feuerstein, G. (1989) *The Yoga-Sutra of Patanjali: A New Translation and Commentary*. Rochester: Inner Traditions International.

Fitzgerald, M. (2011) The neurobiology of chronic pain in children. In: B.C. McClain and S. Suresh, eds. (2011) *Handbook of Pediatric Chronic Pain: Current Science and Integrative Practice*. London: Science+Business Media. Ch. 2.

Fleming, T.M., Merry, S.N., Robinson, E.M., Denny, S.J., & Watson, P.D. (2007) Self-reported suicide attempts and associated risk and protective factors among secondary school students in New Zealand. *Australian and New Zealand Journal of Psychiatry*. 4 (3). p.213–221.

Forbes, B., Akturk, C., Cummer-Nacco, C., Gaither, P., Gotz, J., Harper, A. and Hartsell, K. (2008) Using integrative yoga therapeutics in the treatment of comorbid anxiety and depression. *International Association of Yoga Therapy*. 18. p.87–95.

Forrest, A. (2011) *Fierce Medicine: Breakthrough Practices to Heal the Body and Ignite the Spirit.* New York: HarperCollins Publishing.

Frasier-Thill, R. (2010) Definition of myelination: what myelination means. [online] Available from: http://tweenparenting.about.com/od/physicalemotionalgrowth/a/Definition-of-Myelination.htm [Accessed 28 December 2013].

Gabriels, R.L., Agnew, J.A., Beresford, C., Morrow, M.A., Mesibov, G. & Wamboldt, M. (2012) Improving psychiatric hospital care for pediatric patients with autism spectrum disorders and intellectual disabilities. *Autism Research and Treatment*. 2012 p.1–7.

Galantino, M.L., Galbavy, R. & Quinn, L. (2008) Therapeutic effects of yoga for children: a systematic review of the literature. *Pediatric Physical Therapy.* 20. p.66–80.

Garner, D. (1991) Eating disorder inventory-2: professional manual. Odessa: psychological Assessment Research, Inc.

Gatzounis, R., Schrooten, M.G.S., Crombez, G. & Vlaeyen, J.W.S. (2012) Operant learning theory in pain and chronic pain rehabilitation. *Current Pain Headache Reports.* 16. p.117–126.

Goldberg, L. (2013) *Yoga Therapy for Children with Autism and Special Needs.* New York: W.W. Norton & Company.

Greenberg, M.T. & Harris, A.L. (2011) Nurturing mindfulness in children and youth: current state of research. *Child Development Perspectives.* 6 (2). p.161–166.

Guber, T. & Kalish, L. (2005) *Yoga Pretzels (Yoga Cards).* Bath: Barefoot Books.

Hainsworth, K.R., Salamon, K.S., Khan, K.A., Mascarenbas, B., Davies, W.H. & Weisman, S.J. (2013) A pilot study of yoga for chronic headaches in youth: promise amidst challenges. *Pain Management Nursing*. 15 (2). p.4990–4998.

Hayes, S.C., Strosahl, K.D. & Wilson, K.G. (2003) *Acceptance and Commitment Therapy: An Experiential Approach to Behavior Change.* New York: Guilford.

Heckers, S., Barch, D.M., Bustillo, J., Gaebel, W., Gur, R., Malaspina, D., Owen, M.J., Schultz, S., Tandon, R., Tsuang, M., Van Os, J., and Carpenter, W. (2013) Structure of the psychotic disorders classification in DSM-5. *Schizophrenia Research.* 150. p. 11–14.

Henry (2013) Psychosis is nothing like a badger. [online] Available from: http://www.time-to-change.org.uk/blog/psychosis-nothing-badger [Accessed 8 September 2014].

Herman, J. (1997) *Trauma and Recovery: The Aftermath of Violence—from Domestic Abuse to Political Terror.* New York: Basic Books.

Hiday, V.A., Swartz, M.S., Swanson, J.W., Borum, R., & Wagner, H.R. (1999) Criminal victimization of persons with severe mental illness. *Psychiatric Services*. 50. p. 62–68.

Huber, C.G., Naber, D. & Lambert, M. (2008) Incomplete remission and treatment resistance in first-episode psychosis: definition, prevalence and predictors. [online] Available from: http://informahealthcare.com/doi/abs/10.1517/14656566.9.12.2027 [Accessed 18 August 2014].

Huelke, D.F. (1998) An overview of anatomical considerations of infants and children in the adult world of automobile safety design. *Association for the Advancement of Automotive Medicine.* 42. p.93–113.

International Association of Yoga Therapists. (2014) Contemporary definitions of yoga therapy. [online] Available from http://www.iayt.org/?page=ContemporaryDefinition[Accessed 11 October 2014].

Interlandi, J. (2014) How do you heal a traumatized mind? *The New York Times Magazine.* 25 May, p. 42–47, 52 & 58.

International Association of Yoga Therapists (2014) Contemporary definitions of yoga therapy. [online] Available from http://www.iayt.org/?page=ContemporaryDefinition [Accessed 11 October 2014].

Iyengar, B.K.S. (1979) *Light on Yoga: Revised Edition.* New York: Schocken Books.

Iyengar, B.K.S. (1997) *Light on Pranayama: The Yogic Art of Breathing.* New York: Crossroad.

Iyengar, B.K.S. (2001) *Yoga, the Path to Holistic Healing.* London: Dorling Kindersley.

Joiner, T. (2005) *Why People Die by Suicide.* Cambridge: Harvard University Press.

Kabat-Zinn, J. (1990*) Full Catastrophe Living: Using the Wisdom of Your Body and Mind to Face Stress, Pain, and Illness*. New York: Dell Publishing.

Kaley-Isley, L.C., Peterson, J., Fischer, C. & Peterson, E. (2010) Yoga as a complementary therapy for children and adolescents: a guide for clinicians. *Psychiatry*. 7 (8). p. 20–32.

Kessler, R.C., Aguilar-Gaxiola, S., Alonso, J., Chatterji, S., Lee, S., Ormel, J., Ustun, T.B., & Wang, P.S. (2009) The global burden of mental disorders: an update from the WHO World Mental Health (WMH) surveys. *Epidemiologia e Psichiatria Sociale*. 18 (1). p.23–33.

Klein, J. & Cook-Cottone, C. (2013) The effects of yoga on eating disorder symptoms and correlates; a review. *International Journal of Yoga Therapy*. 23 (2). p. 41–50.

Koerth-Baker, M. (2013) The not-so-hidden causes behind the A.D.H.D. epidemic. *The New York Times.* [online] Available from: http://www.nytimes.com/2013/10/20/magazine/the-not-so-hidden-cause-behind-the-adhd-epidemic.html?pagewanted=all&_r=0 [Accessed 27 September 2014].

Kornfeld, A.B.E. (2009) *Psychotherapy Goes from Couch to Yoga Mat*. [online] Available from: http://content.time.com/time/health/article/0,8599,1891271,00.html [Accessed 2 December 2013].

Kraftsow, G. (1999) *Yoga for Wellness: Healing with the Timeless Teachings of Viniyoga.* New York: Penguin Group.

Kraftsow, G. (2002) *Yoga for Transformation: Ancient Teachings and Practices for Healing the Body, Mind, and Heart.* New York: Penguin Compass.

Lanktree, C. & Briere, J. (2008) Integrative treatment of complex trauma for children (ITCT-C): a guide for the treatment of multiply-traumatized children aged eight to twelve. In: NCTSN (National Children Traumatic Stress Network), *Learning community meeting on integrative treatment of complex trauma.* Long Beach, CA, USA, 22–23 October. Long Beach: MCAVIC.

Levine, P. (1997) *Waking the Tiger—Healing Trauma.* Berkeley: North Atlantic Books.

Lindenboim, N., Comtois, K.A. & Linehan, M. (2007) Skills practice in Dialectical Behavior Therapy for suicidal women meeting criteria for Borderline Personality Disorder. *Cognitive and Behavioural Practice.* 14 (2). p.147–156.

Linehan, M.M., Schmidt, H., Dimeff, L.A., Kanter, J., & Comtois, K.A. (1999) Dialectical Behavior Therapy for patients with Borderline Personality Disorder and drug-dependence. *The American Journal on Addictions.* 8. p. 279–292.

Lock, J. & le Grange, D. (2005) *Help Your Teenager Beat an Eating Disorder.* New York: Guilford Press.

Lu, J.S. & Pierre, J.M. (2007) Letter to the editor: psychotic episode associated with Bikram yoga. *American Journal of Psychiatry.* 164 (11). p.1761.

Mandy, W.P.L., Charman, T. & Skuse, D.H. (2012) Testing the construct validity of proposed criteria for DSM-5 Autism Spectrum Disorder. *Journal of the American Academy of Child and Adolescent Psychiatry.* 51 (1). p.41–50.

Mayo Clinic (2014) What does the research say about food additives and ADHD? [online] Available from: http://www.mayoclinic.org/diseases-conditions/adhd/expert-answers/adhd/faq-20058203 [Accessed 27 September 2014].

McCall, T. (2007) *Yoga as Medicine: The Yogic Prescription for Health and Healing.* New York: Bantam Dell.

McIver, S., McGartland, M., & O'Halloran, P. (2009) Overeating is not about the food: woman describe their experience of yoga treatment program for binge eating. *Qualitative Health Research,* 19 (9). p. 1234–45.

Minshew, N.J. & Goldstein, G. (1998) Autism as a disorder of complex information processing. *Mental Retardation and Developmental Disabilities.* 4. p.129–136.

Namaste Publishing, (2010) I Have Heard So Much about Witnessing State: How Do I Experience It? [online] Available from: http://www.namastepublishing.com/section-5-i-have-heard-so-much-about-witnessing-state-how-do-i-experience-state [Accessed 2 February 2014].

National Association of Anorexia Nervosa and Associated Disorders, (2014) Eating Disorder Statistics. [online] Available from: http://www.anad.org/get-information/about-eating-disorders/eating-disorders-statistics [Accessed 15 May 2014].

National Association of Mental Health (2014) First episodes of psychosis. [online] Available from: www.nami.org/Template.cfm?Section=First_Episode [Accessed 13 September 2014].

National Center for PTSD (2014) Mental health effects of serving in Afghanistan and Iraq. US Department of Veterans Affairs website. [online] Available from: http://www.ptsd.va.gov/public/PTSD-overview/reintegration/overview-mental-health-effects.as [Accessed 1 June 2014].

National Child Traumatic Stress Network (2013) Trauma types. [online] Available from: http://www.nctsn.org/trauma-types [Accessed 28 June 2014].

National Eating Disorder Association (2015) General information: types and symptoms of eating disorders. [online] Available from http:www.nationaleatingdisorders.org/general-information.

National Institute of Mental Health (2013) Bipolar disorder with psychotic features. [online]

Available from: http://psychcentral.com/lib/bipolar-disorder-with-psychotic-features [Accessed 10 September 2014].

National Institute of Neurological Disorders and Stroke (2014) NINDS Pervasive Developmental Disorders Information Page. [online] Available from: http://www.ninds.nih.gov/disorders/pdd/pdd.htm [Accessed 5 October 2014].

Oetzel, K.B. & Scherer, D.G. (2003) Therapeutic engagement with adolescents in psychotherapy. *Psychotherapy: Theory, Research, Practice, Training.* 40 (3). p.215–255.

Ostergaard, S.D. et al. Bertelsen, A., Nielsen, J., Mors, O., and Petrides, G. (2013) The association between psychotic mania, psychotic depression and mixed affective episodes among 14,529 patients with bipolar disorder. *Journal of Affective Disorders*. 147 (1–3). p.44–50.

Partridge, B., Lucke, J. & Hall, W. (2014) Overdiagnosed and overtreated: a survey of Australian public attitudes towards the acceptability of drug treatment for depression and ADHD. [online] Available from: http://www.ncbi.nlm.nih.gov/pmc/articles/PMC3975148/ [Accessed 27 September 2014].

Pearson, N. (2008) Yoga therapy in practice: yoga for people in pain. I*nternational Journal of Yoga Therapy.* 18. p.77–86.

Perry, B.D. (2009) Examining child maltreatment through a neurodevelopmental lens: clinical applications of the neurosequential model of therapeutics. *Journal of Loss and Trauma: International Perspectives on Stress & Coping.* 14 (4). p.240–255.

Piaget, J. (1973) *Main Trends in Psychology.* London: George Allen & Unwin.

Pilkington, K., Kirkwood, G., Rampes, H. & Richardson, J. (2005) Yoga for depression: The research evidence. *Journal of Affective Disorders.* 89. p. 13–24.

Prabhavananda, S. & Isherwood, C. (1981) *How to Know God: The Yoga Aphorisms of Patanjali.* Hollywood: The Vedanta Press.

Prinstein, M.J., Heilbron, N., Guerry, J.D., Franklin, J.C., Rancourt, D., Simon, V., & Spirito, A. (2010) Peer influences and non-suicidal self injury: longitudinal results in community and clinically-referred adolescent samples. *Journal of Abnormal Child Psychology.* 38. p.669–682.

QPR Institute, (2011) What is QPR? [online] Available from http://www.qprinstitute.com/about.html [Accessed 1 September 2014].

Rabiner, D. (2014) *New diagnostic criteria for ADHD.* [online]. Available from: http://www.add.org/?page=DiagnosticCriteria [Accessed 21 September 2014].

Rice University website. (2011) Self-Harm. [online] Available from http://wellbeing.rice.edu/selfharm/ [Accessed 28 July 2014].

Rimland, B. (1964) *Infantile Autism.* New York: Appleton-Century-Crofts.

Rogers, S.J. & Ozonoff, S. (2005) Annotation: What do we know about sensory dysfunction in autism? A critical review of empirical evidence. *Journal of Child Psychology and Psychiatry.* 46 (12). p.1255–1268.

Rogers, S.J. & Vismara, L.A. (2008) Evidence-based comprehensive treatments for early autism. *Journal of Clinical Child and Adolescent Psychology.* 37 (1). p.8–38.

Rothschild, B. (2000) *The Body Remembers: The Psychophysiology of Trauma and Trauma Treatment.* New York: W.W. Norton & Company.

Salmon, P., Lush, E., Jablonski, M. & Sephton, S.E. (2009) Yoga and mindfulness: clinical aspects of an ancient mind/body practice. *Cognitive and Behavioral Practice.* 16. p.59–72.

Santrock, J. (1996) *Child Development.* 13th Edition, Mc Graw Hill Companies.

Saraswati, S.S. (1990) *Yoga Education for Children.* Munger: Yoga Publications Trust.

Schwarz, A. & Cohen, S. (2013) A.D.H.D. seen in 11% of U.S. children as diagnoses rise. [online] Available from: http://www.nytimes.com/2013/04/01/health/more-diagnoses-of-hyperactivity-causing-concern.

html?pagewanted=all&_r=0 [Accessed 26 September 2014].

Scime, M., & Cook-Cottone, C. (2008) Primary prevention of eating disorders: A constructivist integration of mind and body strategies. *International Journal of Eating Disorders*. 41 (2) 4. p. 134–42.

Serani, D. (2012) Depression and non-suicidal self injury. [online] Available from: http://www.psychologytoday.com/blog/two-takes-depression/201202/depression-and-non-suicidal-self-injury [Accessed 28 July 2014].

Shapiro, D., & Cline, K. (2004) Mood changes associated with Iyengar Yoga practices: A pilot study. *International Association of Yoga Therapy*. 14. p. 35–44.

Sheean, L. (2010) Thinking about suicide: contemplating and comprehending the urge to die. [online] Available from: http://youthfocus.com.au/wp-content/uploads/2011/02/David-Webb-article1.pdf [Accessed 5 August 2014].

Siegel, M. & Gabriels, R.L. (2014) Psychiatric hospital treatment of children with autism and serious behavioral disturbance. *Child Adolescent Psychiatric Clinics of North America*. 23. p.125–142.

Singer, D.G. & Revenson, T.A. (1997) *A Piaget Primer: How a Child Thinks* (Revised Edition). Madison: International Universities Press, Inc.

Spinazzola, J., Rhodes, A.M., Emerson, D., Earle, E., & Monroe, K. (2011) Application of yoga in residential treatment of traumatized youth. *Journal of American Psychiatric Nurses Association*. 17 (6). p.431–444.

Steiner, H., Kwan, W., Shaffer, T.G., Walker, S., Miller, S., Sagar, A., & Lock, J. (2003) Risk and protective factors for juvenile eating disorders. *European Child & Adolescent Psychiatry*. 1 (12). p.38–46.

Streeter, C., Jensen, J.E., Perlmutter, R.M., Cabral, H.J., Tian, J., Terhune, D.B., Ciraulo, D.A., & Renshaw, P.F. (2007) Yoga asana sessions increase brain GABA levels: A pilot study. *The Journal of Alternative and Complementary Medicine*. 13 (4). p. 419–426.

Stuart, H. (2003) Violence and mental illness: an overview. *World Psychiatry*. 2 (2). p.121–124.

Taylor, P.J. (2008) Psychosis and violence: stories, fears, and reality. *The Canadian Journal of Psychiatry*. 53 (10). p.647–659.

Therapeutic Recreation/Child Life & Nursing Education Departments (1990) *Growth and development summary*. Aurora: Children's Hospital Colorado.

Tracey, I. (2010) Getting the pain you expect: mechanisms of placebo, nocebo and reappraisal effects in humans. *Nature Medicine*. 16 (11). p.1277–1283.

Tylka, T.L. (2004) The relation between body dissatisfaction and eating disorder symptomatology: an analysis of moderating variable. *Journal of Counseling Psychology*, 51(2). p. 178–191.

Vadiraja, S. H., Rao, M.R., Nagendra, R.H., Nagartha, R., Rehka, M., Vanitha, N., Gopinath, S.K., Srinath, B.S, Vishweshwara, M.S., Madhavi, Y.S., Ajaikumar, B.S, Ramesh, S.B., & Rao, N. (2009) Effects of yoga on symptom management in breast cancer patients: a randomized controlled trial. *International Journal of Yoga*. 2 (2). p.73– 79.

van der Kolk, B. A. (1994) The body keeps score: memory and the evolving psychobiology of post traumatic stress. *Harvard Review of Psychiatry*. 1 (5). p. 253– 265.

van der Kolk, B. A. (2003) Neurobiology of childhood trauma and abuse. *Child and Adolescent Psychiatric Clinics*. 12. p.293–317.

van der Kolk, B.A. (2009) Yoga and post-traumatic stress disorder: an interview with Bessel van der Kolk, MD. Integral Yoga Magazine. Summer Issue. p.12–13.

Viggiano, E., 2014. An interview and conversation with Erica Viggiano. Interviewed by Michelle J. Fury. [iPhone5/voice memo] Denver, CO, USA, 18 July 2014, Appendix.

Walsh, B. (2012) *Treating Self-Injury*. Second Edition. New York: The Guilford Press.

Weintraub, A. (2013) The two-way street: integrating yoga into mental healthcare and mood management into yoga therapy. *International Association of Yoga Therapy*. 9(3). p. 16–18.

Western University website (2013) Self Harm. [online] Available from: http://www.health.uwo.ca/services/students/encyclopedia/self_harm.html [Accessed 28 July 2014].

Winnicott, D.W. (1965) *The Maturational Processes and the Facilitating Environment: Studies in the Theory of Emotional Development*. London: Karnac Books.

Winnicott, D.W. (1971) *Playing and Reality*. London: Tavistock Publications.

Woolery, A., Myers, J., Sternlieg B., & Zeltzer, L. (2004) A yoga intervention for young adults with elevated symptoms of depression. *Alternative Therapies in Health and Medicine*. 10(2). p. 60–63.

World Health Organization website, (2013) *Question and answer about autistic spectrum disorder (ASD)*. [online]. Available from: http://www.who.int/features/qa/85/en/ [Accessed 21 September 2014].

Wren, A.A., Wright, M.A., Carson, J.W., & Keefe, F.J. (2010) Yoga for persistent pain: New findings and directions for an ancient practice. *Pain*. 152. p. 477–480.

Zajac, A.U., & Schier, K. (2011). Body image dysphoria and motivation to exercise: a study of Canadian and Polish women participating in yoga or aerobics. *Archives of Psychiatry and Psychother apy*. 4. p. 67–72.

Zernikow, B., Wager, J. Hechler, T., Sasan, C., Rohr, U., Dobe, M., Meyer, A., Hubner-Mohler, B., Wansler, C., & Blankenburg, M. (2012) Characteristics of highly impaired children with severe chronic pain: a 5-year old retrospective study on 2249 pediatric pain patients. [online] Available from http://biomedcentral.com/1471-2431/12/54 [Accessed 16 December 2014].

Appendix

Transcript of Interview and Conversation with Erica Viggiano 18 July 2014

Erica Viggiano, LCSW, RDN, CACIII, E-RYT, is the creator and director of Integrative Life Services (ILS), which offers integrative health services, including mindfulness and yoga based psychotherapy, life and mindful eating coaching, counseling and other evidence based services. ILS has a contract with the State of Colorado to provide services to adolescents and families in the juvenile justice system.

Viggiano has created Mind Body Self Regulation Yoga™ (MBSR Yoga), a manualized somatic psychotherapy intervention rooted in the traditions of hatha yoga and other mindful awareness practices. Using a neurobiological understanding of trauma symptoms, the model was developed to target psycho-physiological difficulties in self-regulation associated with PTSD and complex trauma. As a clinical intervention, MBSR Yoga has been implemented over the last seven years in child welfare, juvenile justice, residential, home, community and outpatient settings. It is a trauma-focused approach that can also address co-occurring and somatically based challenges, such as substance abuse, compulsive or binge eating, aggression and self-harm. Subjects in a pilot study reported that they used skills outside of intervention sessions to manage stress more effectively.

MJF: When did you establish Integrative Life Services?

EV: In 2001 or 2003 I started doing a fair amount of yoga and mindfulness based clinical work. I had been doing training and various evidence based practices through ILS for a while. Around that time I completed my yoga teacher training and started creating opportunities to work primarily in that modality (of Integrative Life Services).

MJF: I love the way you put that: yoga and mindfulness based clinical services.

EV: Yes, yoga and mindfulness psychotherapy. That's the primary focus of what we do. (We also specialize in) trauma intervention for adults and adolescents, as well as treating binge and compulsive eating. There are a variety of mood challenges that go with both of those problems, including addiction. So addiction is another focus. I see the addiction focus as something that needs specialized attention. But it's often part of healing from trauma and from binge eating, whether it's substance addiction or other kinds of addictions. The company has been a wonderful opportunity to work with a variety of different groups. These include private practice clients, workshops for yoga and mindfulness to address binge eating and trauma, as well as youth and families involved in the juvenile justice system, who may not have the financial access for those sorts of services. So it's a real gift to have a contract with the State of Colorado, and the means to make these services accessible to them—whether they're (receiving services) in the community, or while they're still in a locked facility, or in the home.

For instance, I first met a client at a child welfare placement. He's now in the youth corrections system, and unfortunately has a common story. He has not committed a lot of crimes. But as a result of his trauma he has a lot of problems with self-regulation. And unsupported and untreated, he's assaulted some people. Now he's a 19-year-old in the division of youth corrections. Through that contract, I have the opportunity to help him connect with a yoga class that fits for him, and that is financially accessible to him. So we found a studio that is a true donation studio, and he's budgeting his money so he can pay three dollars a class.

MJF: Are you his primary therapist?

EV: No, in this case I'm helping him (find yoga services). I've known him for three years from teaching yoga therapy to him when he was in the residential placement. I can interface with his primary therapist if needed. But often it's not needed because he's at the point where he knows what he needs, and he's asked for support in doing this for himself.

MJF: Earlier in his treatment were you more involved in talking or collaborating with the primary therapist?

EV: Not in this case . . . in some cases I do individual yoga and mindfulness based therapy that includes a direct focus on trauma and some kind of exposure therapy. Other times, if it's agreed that primarily self-regulation skills, affect tolerance, affect management skills are most needed for the young person I would be doing that work. But if the client does have another primary therapist, I'd be collaborating with the therapist. I do that a lot with other therapists throughout the juvenile justice system. So I work as a primary therapist. But sometimes I work as an adjunct therapist.

MJF: So you're part of the trauma team, and you're involved in the comprehensive trauma treatment?

EV: Yes, sometimes I am the trauma therapist. Sometimes I'm doing the mind-body self-regulation. And either way, it's both possible and important to be communicating really closely with any other therapist who's involved.

I do notice that some therapists who may not have a lot of experience with trauma often don't understand (or are not able to track) the level of activation that goes on when they engage clients in talking about aspects of their trauma.

MJF: How do you track that?

EV: I often start by my own observation as a clinician. I pay a great deal of attention to physiological cues that someone might be experiencing sympathetic arousal—breath, flushing in the face, rigid body posture, talking fast, talking slow . . .

MJF: A change in the cadence of their speech?

EV: Yes, a change in cadence, a change in breath, a change in the way you can see someone's skin flush when they talk about certain things. Or, on the other side, hypo-arousal—just seeing a client get quiet, distant, or her mind seems to be going somewhere else. Fairly quickly I try to help clients build enough awareness to have the language for communicating with me. For instance, being able to say, "I felt my breath get really fast," or, "My mind started going somewhere else." So whether we're primarily talking or we're doing physical practices, there begins to be this emerging practice of staying checked in with each other, using both observation and language to communicate what's going on physiologically.

MJF: What you said there is so critical—that regardless of whether you're doing yoga therapy or doing talk therapy, you're always tracking the body's experience, and the changes you and the client notice. It sounds like you're a mirror to help them become more aware of tracking.

EV: I think of it as a kind of co-regulation. We often talk about co-regulation when we talk about parents being attuned to their children as they're growing and developing. As therapists, I see us as co-regulating with the client and partnering so that ultimately the client is really skilled at recognizing. That's the endgame—like you said, you're helping mirror back for them what's happening. Even if they suddenly want to tell you a lot, you can check in with them. Not telling them what to say or not to say, you can instead ask, "What's happening right now? What are you feeling? What do you feel in your breath? What are you feeling in your body? What do you want to do next? Should we keep talking about this? Or would you like to do something that slows your body down a little bit? What would feel best right now?"

MJF: You're helping the client regulate. You're increasing his awareness, and he gets to make the decision. Just now you've talked about so much. In some ways you're helping re-parent. But you're also teaching the client to parent himself, and you're mirroring him, which we know is so important in attachment theory. But the mirroring may have either never happened or happened incompletely.

EV: As we know from child development, most of what's happening developmentally is both physical and physiological. It's a physical symbiosis.

MJF: They don't have the words yet.

EV: Right, it's not any kind of verbal attunement. It's that part of both of our brains that's really tuned in to what we're feeling now. I don't know if you notice this, but after a while I feel it in my body a lot more when someone is starting to get hyper-aroused, or even starting to check out.

MJF: Dissociating . . .

EV: Yes, getting quiet, and literally going some place else in their mind. (Attuning with the client) not only helps me as a clinician, it also helps me take care of myself. Interestingly enough, even with a fair amount of trauma work and severe traumatic experiences in a lot of my clients, I don't find myself feeling burnt out, depleted or drained.

MJF: You've mentioned that tracking your own experience during the session helps you. Are there things you do before and after that also help you self-regulate?

EV: The foundation we're operating on is that being attuned to somebody and being connected with them doesn't mean you have to take on their emotions. There's a way to just be present, and to recognize that their experience is not my experience. I think what I do before a session is that I make sure that I'm really grounded. By holding a boundary, you're connected but you're also separate.

MJF: I'd like to touch on two terms—complex trauma and developmental trauma, neither of which is used in the DSM-5. It seems like complex trauma is the term initially used when (our field) realized there's something more than PTSD. But now we understand it's developmental, so developmental trauma is the newer term.

EV: I think so. It's complex because it's occurred throughout a child's development. It's occurred during pivotal stages of development. (Those who suffer developmental trauma) are missing a lot of the basic building blocks that help people cope, help people feel safe in the world, and help people feel like they're effective in the world. My belief is that there are a lot of misdiagnosed people out there who have experienced developmental trauma throughout their lives. Now they're in their twenties, or they're in their thirties, but they're being (diagnosed with) Borderline Personality Disorder, because they're having a difficult time coping.

When I think about combat veterans and combat PTSD, the vets' attachment history has a lot to do with how resilient they're going to be. So if they had relatively secure attachments, they're not necessarily going to be as vulnerable to traumatic events. Even if there is PTSD that emerges as a result of their combat experiences, it might be shorter term if they receive the right treatment matched to their situation. But for somebody who has experienced insecure attachment through a great deal of his childhood and early adolescence, he's going to react to trauma that occurs later on in life much differently, and perhaps with less resilience.

MJF: What you're saying is that these two vets can both have PTSD. But the one who had insecure attachment, and then has combat trauma, may experience developmental trauma. He might be much more profoundly traumatized by war.

EV: Yes, because of the unmet developmental needs, the person doesn't have as many developmental tools to withstand an assault on the senses, and an assault on his experience.

MJF: . . . And an assault on the self.

EV: Yes, on the sense of self, that's a good way to put it.

MJF: You've said something to me before about clients who experience developmental trauma by being shamed. So that's what happens—developmental trauma occurs when one doesn't develop a full sense of self. Thus, when one sees the horrors of war, it's going to be a bigger assault on one's sense of self if one did have insecure attachment.

EV: Yes, it occurs to me that what I was describing about those clients who experience such a severely humiliating or shaming experience, is that they carry it with them the way one might carry the experience of rape or sexual abuse. It's a lot more likely that it's going to happen with someone who has developmental trauma, whether it was an insensitive parent or an insensitive environment or insecure attachment to begin with. Humiliation can be experienced as something that shatters the sense of self, shatters the sense of "I'm ok, and I'm going to be taken care of." Oftentimes trauma comes from a life-threatening experience, but other times it's an almost life-threatening assault to the sense of self.

MJF: This may be what's behind the movement to codify the term developmental trauma. It's not just that a person perceives that he could be killed, it's that his sense of self is feeling threatened. And when the sense of self feels like it could be annihilated, that's traumatic. If it happens at a young age, then one hasn't developed a sense of self yet fully.

EV: In early development, when you perceive your mother as being removed—whether it's her rejecting you or you being taken out of her home and put in foster care—at that stage of development it is an annihilation of the self. One has no other way of feeling secure in the world, and one doesn't exist as a self without that connection to a primary caregiver. So it is annihilation. I like that word, because it is a sense of annihilation to the integrity of self, the integrity of who I am, the integrity of having my basic needs met.

MJF: And mirror, someone to mirror your experience.

EV: And someone to say it's going to be ok, and you believe them. That does not happen for children who grow up in homes that are so chaotic where their attachment relationships are not secure. Any experience that creates a sense of annihilation or severe threat to the integrity of the self can cause trauma. I think it's misunderstood within the field. It's one of the reasons that people go to the hospital and get diagnosed with a bunch of symptoms before (a medical provider) thinks about whether the individual has experienced such significant trauma that she's really depressed . . . or has obsessive compulsive disorder along with it, or is cutting along with it, or substance abuse due to the trauma. But for someone not trained in trauma, assessing for trauma literally becomes an after thought.

MJF: It is an after thought.

EV: Trauma really needs to be assessed throughout treatment.

Index

[Index to: Yoga Therapy/Children (Handspring Mar 2015)]

A

abdominal (stomach) migraines, 27, 38
Acceptance and Commitment Therapy, 37
action-oriented techniques in
  psychosis, 77, 79
adaptations in development, 5–8
Adho Mukha Svanasana (Downward-facing Dog), 30, 31, 48, 85, 88–9, 104
adolescents (15–18 years), 7–8
  breathing techniques, 87–8
  eating disorders, 60–1
  mood regulation, 32–6
  pain, 12–13
  psychosis, 79
  self-injury, 71–3
  suicidal ideation, 69–70
  trauma symptoms, 47–9
  visualization and relaxation exercises, 110–11
age and development, 5–8
ahimsa (non-violence), 62
Airplane Pose (Virabhadrasana III), 70, 72, 91–2
annihilation of the self, 38, 124
anorexia nervosa, 52, 55
anxiety
  case study, 26
  practice for adolescents, 33–4
anxiety disorders, 21
Apanasana Vinyasa, 16, 18, 89
arousal *see* hyper-arousal; hypo-arousal
asanas (poses/postures), 11, 23, 88–111
  adolescent, 8
  see also specific poses
attention deficit hyperactivity disorder (ADHD), 81, 83, 84, 85
attention issues (in general), 84–5
autistic spectrum disorder (ASD), 81–5
autonomic nervous system, 41

B

Baddha Konasana (Bound Angle/Cobbler's Pose) A, 15, 34, 36, 49, 80, 89–90
Baddha Konasana (Bound Angle/Cobbler's Pose) B, 34, 36, 90
Balasana (Child's Pose; Rock Pose), 4, 15, 17, 19, 30, 31, 47, 48, 70, 73, 80, 85, 86, 90–1, 104
  case study, 44
  modifications, 90
Balloon Breath, 87
bare attention, 24
behavioral health issues
  PTSD, 39
  suicidal ideation and self-injury, 68
behavioral regulation, 21–36
bell curve versus individual, 8
Bhujangasana (Cobra Pose), 1, 15, 30, 32, 47, 70, 86, 91, 104
  modification (Sphinx Pose), 91, 104
binge eating, 121
  and purging, 52
binge eating disorder, 52
biopsychosocial nature of pain, 11–12
  see also neurobiology
bipolar disorder
  case study, 10, 27–8
  psychosis and, 76, 77, 78
Birthday Candle Breath, 87
Boat Pose (Paripurna Navasana), 72, 80, 96
body image issues and body awareness, 51–9
Bound Angle Pose *see* Baddha Konasana
Box Breathing, 87
boy with eating disorder, 59
brain
  autistic spectrum disorder and, 81
  development and neuroplasticity, 3–4
  myelination, 7, 17
breathing techniques, 87–8
  Counting Breaths, 18, 47, 49, 61, 71, 87–9
  Snake Breath, 4, 6, 10, 15, 16, 29, 30, 31, 61, 85, 88
  viloma Breathing/pranayama, 67, 88
  see also Green Breath meditation
Bridge Pose (Setu Bandha Sarvangasana), 16, 18, 36, 69, 72, 80, 100–1
bulimia nervosa, 52, 55

C

Candlestick Pose (Salamba Sarvangasana Variation), 100, 107
Chicken Wing (Gomukhasana Arms), 18, 93
chronic pain, 11–19
Cobbler's Pose *see* Baddha Konasana
Cobra Pose *see* Bhujangasana
cognitive functioning
  adolescents, 7
  pre-schoolers, 6
  psychosis and, 77
  school-agers, 7
  slow cognitive processing, 81, 84
concrete thinking, 7
constrictive symptoms of trauma, 40
copycat behavior, suicidal ideation and self-injurious behavior, 67
Corpse Pose (Relaxation Pose; Savasana), 17, 19, 30, 32, 34, 61, 70, 86, 99–100
Counting Breaths, 18, 47, 49, 61, 71, 87–8
Creative Relaxation®, 84
Criss-Cross Apple Sauce (Sukhasana; Simple Sitting Pose), 15, 16, 18, 30, 31, 35, 36, 46, 47, 49, 61, 69, 71, 85, 101–2, 105
cystic fibrosis (CF), 13–14

D

delusions, 76, 77
depression
  case study, 26
  practice for adolescents, 34–6
  psychosis and, 77
  suicidal ideation and, 67
development, 3–9
  rules of conduct and, 2
  trauma in and affecting, 40, 123, 124
dialectic of trauma, Herman's, 40, 42, 45
Dikasana B (Airplane Pose; Virabhadrasana III), 70, 72, 91–2
Downward-facing Dog (Adho Mukha Svanasana), 30, 31, 48, 85, 88–9, 104
Dynamic Bridge Pose (Setu Bandha Sarvangasana), 16, 18, 36, 72, 80, 100–1

E

Eagle Pose (Garudasana), 32, 34, 92–3
Ear-of-the-Cow Arms (Chicken Wing; Gomukhasana Arms), 18, 93
early interventions (in life), 3
  attention deficit hyperactivity disorder, 83
eating disorders, 51–62
  case studies, 43–4, 57–9
  defining, 51–2
  practice considerations, 59–61
  risk and protective factors, 53–6
egotism, 6
Eka Pada Rajakapotasana prep (Pigeon Pose), 34, 36, 61, 80, 92
emotions, 21–36
  avoiding, 24
  eating disorders and awareness of, 55
  eating disorders and regulation of, 55–6, 57–8
  non-attachment to, 26
  recognizing and accepting, 24–6
empathy in family system, 62
Extended Side Angle Pose (Side Angle Stretch; Utthita Parsvakonasana), 48, 106
Extended Triangle (Utthita Trikonasana), 70, 76, 106–7
Eye of the Needle Pose (Sucirandhra), 47, 49, 61, 101

F

family (and family system)
  eating disorder treatment and, 52–3, 62
  empathy, 62
  system, 9
  see also multifamily group therapy

Feuerstein, Georg, 1, 2, 23
fight–flight–freeze response, 41
Five-Minute Vacation, 32, 110
Forward Fold Straddle (Prasarita Padottanasana A; Wide Legged Forward Fold), 61, 98–9

G

Garudasana (Eagle Pose), 32, 34, 92–3
Goldberg, Louise, 82, 83, 84–5
Gomukhasana Arms (Chicken-Wing; Ear-of-the-Cow Arms), 18, 93
Green Breath meditation, 61, 110
group therapy in eating disorders, multifamily, 51, 60, 62

H

hallucinations, 29, 75, 76, 77
Hamstring Stretch, 93–4
Hastasana (Waterfall Pose), 16, 18, 94
Head-to-Knee Pose (Janu Sirsasana), 16, 18, 49, 72, 94–5
headache, 11, 12, 19, 27
Herman's dialectic of trauma, 40, 42, 45
holding environment, 23–4
hyper-arousal, 40, 41, 82
hypo-arousal, 81, 82, 122

I

individual versus bell curve, 8
injuries
    self-inflicted, 63–73
    sports, 8, 32
integrated (multidisciplinary team) care, 28, 29
    suicidal ideation and self-injurious behavior, 64
Integrative Life Services (ILS), 121
Integrative Yoga Therapeutics®, 68
Intense Side Stretch (Pyramid Pose; Parsvottanasana), 80, 97
International Association of Yoga Therapy (IAYT), 2, 8
intrusive symptoms of trauma, 40
Iyengar, B.K.S., 1, 2, 11, 21, 67, 78

J

Janu Sirsasana (Head-to-Knee/Runner's Stretch Pose), 16, 18, 49, 72, 94–5

K

Knees to Chest Pose (Apanasana Vinyasa), 16, 18, 89

L

Legs-up-the-Wall Pose (Viparita Karani), 15, 17, 19, 107
LifeForce Yoga®, 68
Lunge, 31, 34, 46, 48, 69, 79, 95

M

magical thinking, 6
mania, 77
Marichyasana C or modification, 18, 95–6
masculine perspective of eating disorders, 59
meditation, 24
    Green Breath, 61, 110
    psychosis and, 78, 79
    see also mindfulness
memories, traumatic, neurobiology, 38–9
mental health/psychological problems and disorders (in general), 8–9, 22–36
    case study, 10
    chronic pain-related, 12
    global burden, 21, 23, 28
    see also specific disorders
migraines, stomach, 27, 38
Mind Body Self Regulation Yoga™ (MBSR Yoga), 121
mindfulness/mindful awareness, 24, 43, 121
    see also meditation
mood regulation
    abnormal (dysregulation and fluctuations), 21–2, 24, 25, 67, 68, 68–9
    practices, 29–36
Mountain Pose (Tadasana), 16, 18, 30, 46, 48, 60, 86, 91, 92, 93, 94, 97, 98, 105, 106, 108, 109
multidisciplinary care *see* integrated care
multifamily group therapy in eating disorders, 51, 60, 62
myelination, 7, 17

N

National Child Traumatic Stress Network, 40, 43, 45
nervous system
    trauma and, 40, 41
    yoga for psychosis and, 77, 79
neurobiology of traumatic memories, 38–9, 39
neuroplasticity, 3–4
niyamas, 2
non-suicidal self-injury, 63–73

O

obesity, 52, 55
obstacle course intervention in eating disorders, 62
Ocean Breath, 88
One-Footed Royal Pigeon Pose (Eka Pada Rajakapotasana prep), 34, 36, 61, 80, 92
overweight/obesity, 52, 55

P

pain, chronic, 11–19
parasympathetic nervous system, 41
Paripurna Navasana (Boat Pose), 72, 80, 96
Parivrtta Trikonasana (Reverse Triangle), 72, 96–7
Parsvottanasana (Pyramid Pose), 80, 97
Paschimottanasana (Seated Forward Fold), 32, 34, 36, 49, 61, 97–8
Patanjali, 1–2, 23, 26
Peaceful Warrior *see* Virabhadrasana
personality disorder, 75, 123
physical health and psychosis, 77
Pigeon Pose (Eka Pada Rajakapotasana prep), 34, 36, 61, 80, 92
Plank, 98
    see also Upward Plank
poses *see* asanas
post-traumatic stress disorder *see* trauma
Prasarita Padottanasana A (Wide Legged Forward Fold), 61, 98–9
pre-operational stage in development, 6
pre-school child (3-5 years), 6–7
    breathing techniques, 87, 88
    chronic pain, 14–15
    mood regulation, 29
psychological problems *see* mental health problems; trauma
psychology of pain, 12–13
psychopathy, 75
psychosis, 75–80
    contraindications, 78
    myths and mastery, 75–6
    practice considerations, 79–80
Purvottanasana (Upward Plank Pose), 34, 36, 99
Pyramid Pose (Parsvottanasana), 80, 97

Q

QPR (Question Persuade and Refer), 68

R

randomized controlled trials, 2–3, 8, 22
    eating disorders, 53, 56, 59
    psychosis, 76, 77
rapport, 8, 9
Reclining Big Toe Pose (Supine Leg Stretch; Supta Padangusthasana), 32, 34, 103
relaxation exercises, 110–11
Relaxation Pose (Corpse Pose; Savasana), 17, 19, 30, 32, 34, 61, 70, 86, 99–100

research, 2–3
see also randomized controlled trials
Reverse/Revolved Triangle (Parivrtta Trikonasana), 72, 96–7
Rothschild's braking and accelerating metaphor, 42–3
rules of conduct, 2
Runner's Stretch (Hamstring Stretch), 93–4
Runner's Stretch (Janu Sirsasana), 16, 18, 49, 72, 94–5

S

Sa Ta Na Ma mantra, 36, 47, 49, 67, 73, 77, 79, 100, 103, 110–11
Salamba Sarvangasana Variation, 100, 107
satya (speaking the truth), 62
Savasana (Relaxation Pose), 17, 19, 30, 32, 34, 61, 70, 86, 99–100
schizophrenia, 3, 75, 76, 77, 78
school-aged child (5-13 years), 7
breathing techniques, 87–8
chronic pain, 16–17
mood regulation, 29–32
relaxation exercise, 111
trauma symptoms, 46–7
scope of practice, 8–9
Seated Forward Fold (Paschimottanasana), 32, 34, 36, 49, 61, 97–8
Seated Twist (Marichyasana C or modification), 18, 95–6
Seated Twist (Sukhasana Twist), 102
Seated Wide-Angle Pose, 15, 32, 105
self-annihilation, 38, 124
self-competence and eating disorders, 53, 55, 57–8
self-esteem and eating disorders, 53, 56
self-injury, 63–73
self-objectification and eating disorders, 54
sensory integration issues, 81–6
Setu Bandha Sarvangasana (Bridge Pose), 16, 18, 36, 69, 72, 80, 100–1
Side Angle Stretch (Utthita Parsvakonasana), 48, 106
Simple Sitting Pose (Sukasana), 15, 16, 18, 30, 31, 35, 46, 47, 61, 69, 71, 85, 101–2, 105
Skills Training in Affective and Interpersonal Regulation (STAIR) model, 45–6
Snake Breath, 4, 6, 10, 15, 16, 29, 30, 31, 61, 85, 88
social life and chronic pain, 13
special needs, 83, 84–5
Sphinx Pose, 91, 104
sports injury, 8, 32
STAIR (Skills Training in Affective and Interpersonal Regulation) model, 45–6
stomach migraines, 27, 38
stress and psychosis, 77
Sucirandhra (Eye of the Needle Pose), 47, 49, 61, 101
suicidal ideation, 63–73
Sukhasana (Simple Sitting Pose), 15, 16, 18, 30, 31, 35, 36, 46, 47, 49, 61, 69, 71, 85, 101–2, 105
Sukhasana Twist, 102
Sun Salutation (Surya Namaskar), 27, 33, 34, 35, 60, 71, 104
Supine Leg Stretch (Supta Padangusthasana), 32, 34, 103
Supported (Passive) Backbend, 102–3
Supported Shoulderstand (Salamba Sarvangasana) Variation, 100, 107
Supta Padangusthasana (Supine Leg Stretch), 32, 34, 103
Surya Namaskar (Sun Salutation), 27, 33, 34, 35, 60, 71, 104
svadhayaya (study of the self), 2, 62
sympathetic nervous system, 41

T

Tadasana (Mountain Pose), 16, 18, 30, 46, 48, 60, 86, 91, 92, 93, 94, 97, 98, 105, 106, 108, 109
TEACCH (Treatment and Education of Autistic and related Communication Handicapped Children) model, 84, 85
team (integrated) care, 28
team care see integrated care
10 Golden Rules (Goldberg's), 85
thinness, eating disorders and the drive for, 54
training, suicide prevention, 67–8
trauma (psychological incl. post-traumatic stress disorder/PTSD), 37–49
adult vs. childhood experience, 39–40
definitions, 38
development and, 40, 123, 124
memories of, neurobiology, 38–9
practice considerations, 45–9
suicidal ideation and, 67
Viggiano (Erica) on, 121–4
Tree Pose (Vrksasana), 6, 32, 33, 36, 46, 49, 61, 63, 64, 70, 72, 80, 86, 109
Triangle (Utthita Trikonasana), 70, 76, 106–7
see also Reverse Triangle

U

Upavistha Konasana (Seated Wide-Angle Pose), 15, 32, 105
Upward Plank Pose (Purvottanasana), 34, 36, 99
Utthita Parsvakonasana (Side Angle Stretch), 48, 106
Utthita Trikonasana (Triangle), 70, 76, 106–7

V

Viggiano, Erica, interview and conversation with, 121–4
viloma Breathing/pranayama, 67, 88
Viparita Karani (Legs-up-the-Wall Pose), 15, 17, 19, 107
Virabhadrasana I (Warrior/Peaceful Warrior I), 31, 33, 48, 70, 72, 79, 86, 108
Virabhadrasana II (Warrior/Peaceful Warrior II), 30, 31, 33, 46, 48, 61, 70, 72, 79, 108–9
Virabhadrasana III (Warrior III/Airplane Pose), 70, 72, 91–2
visual schedules, 84
Visualizations, 110–11
Green Breath, 61, 110
Vrksasana (Tree Pose), 6, 32, 33, 36, 46, 49, 61, 63, 64, 70, 72, 80, 86, 109

W

Warrior see Virabhadrasana
Waterfall Pose (Hastasana), 16, 18, 94
weight-loss, eating disorders and the motivation for, 54
Weintraub, Amy, 9, 68
Wide Legged Forward Fold (Prasarita Padottanasana A), 61, 98–9
Wide-Angle (Seated) Pose, 15, 32, 105
Windshield Wipers Pose, 34, 70, 86, 109–10
Winnicott, Donald, 1, 2, 23–4, 25

Y

yoga (and yoga therapy), basics, 1–3
Yoga Nidra, 34, 70, 73, 111
Yoga Pretzels®, 62, 84